How to Lose Water Weight

The Fastest Way to Flush

Out 20 Pounds in 30 Days

By Camille Hugh

Also by Camille Hugh

The Thigh Gap Hack

Bye-Bye Thunder Thighs

The Skinny Girl Bible

The Oil-Free Diet

Your Free Gift

I'd like to reward you with a FREE sneak peek access to my new workout DVD "CARDIOTWIST". It is a one hour long video that combines the absolute best twisting and fluid draining moves from yoga along with a cardio flow that will keep your heart beating, body sweating and target fat burning.

This video is the perfect complement to this book and will give you the ability to jump head first into your weight loss plan as soon as you finished reading.

To find out more information and sign up, visit www.thighgaphack.com and enter your name and email on the very top of the page.

Note to Readers

The content of this book, by its very nature, is general, whereas each reader's situation is unique. Therefore, the purpose is to provide general information rather than to address individual situations.

This book proposes a program of diet and exercise based on the opinions and ideas of the author. It is intended to provide helpful and informative material on the subject addressed in the publication and is sold with the understanding that the author and publisher are not engaged in rendering medical, health, psychological, or any other kind of personal professional services or therapy in the book.

The reader should consult his or her qualified medical, health, psychological, or other competent professional before starting this or any other fitness program, particularly if you suffer from any medical condition or have any symptom that may require treatment.

If at any time you experience any discomfort, stop immediately and consult your physician. The author and publisher specifically disclaim all responsibility for any liability, loss, or risk, personal or otherwise, which is incurred as a consequence, directly or indirectly, of the use and application of any of the contents of this book.

Published in the United Stated by The Feminine Contour, LLC

www.thighgaphack.com

CONTENTS

INTRODUCTION

What do wrestlers, ballet dancers, strength athletes (body builders, Olympic lifters, power lifters, cross fitters), bikini and runway models, weight loss game show contestants, and ultimate fighters have in common? The answer lies is weight cutting or more specifically, the ability to lose a tremendous amount of weight (up to 20 pounds) in a relatively short period of time – we are talking days and weeks.

I am fully aware the claims of losing twenty pounds in a matter of days seems like the hogwash fodder late night infomercials are made of and way too good to be true, but I exaggerate and kid you not. Every year thousands of individuals accomplish seemingly impossible weight loss and they do it all for a leg up on their competition or to earn a paycheck.

It is no secret weight can play a major role in who wins or loses a match or even a job position. For example, in combat sports, those who weigh more obviously have the upper hand, so it is a well known tactic for competitors to lose a ton of weight fast so they can qualify for lower weight classes and then put the weight back on very quickly so that they can be significantly bigger than their opponents.

On the opposite end of the spectrum, for other sports or careers like equestrian riders, weighing as little as possible makes all the difference. Think of the weight loss television competition *'The Biggest Loser'*, where millions of dollars are up for grabs simply for the person who is able to lose the largest amount of weight in a very short time. Any trick that will contribute to the number on the scale dipping lower will undoubtedly be exploited.

Now, what is a lesser-known fact is how these athletes, every day people and models manage to actually drop the weight. I can tell you right now that eating right and exercising for a few days or weeks won't lead to such drastic results. Yes, it is the healthy way to drop the pounds but it is not the only or even nearly the most expeditious way, and while a common misconception is that fat loss is the only culprit for the slim bodies these individuals display, the truth is it's not.

You see, proper diet and exercise goes hand in hand with slow and steady weight loss. In fact, the guidelines for safe fat loss are only one to two pounds per week - a far cry from the twenty to thirty pounds (the larger you are the more you can lose) some of these folks can lose in a few days. So, what gives?

Water, that's what. Believe it or not, the drastic weight loss is not fat or adipose tissue, but water. According to the United States Geology Survey, the human body is made up of sixty to seventy percent water. Water, along with your organs, fat, tissue, etc. all contribute to the number that greets you when you step on the scale and also has a lot to do with your appearance. Just think about how your stomach looks when you are bloated or have just finished eating a carb heavy meal versus how it looks when you wake up first thing in the morning.

CAN YOU LOSE WATER WEIGHT?

Given the make up of our bodies I can say without a doubt that the majority of weight you are carrying right now is because of water weight, and a great deal of you reading this will have excess water retention beyond typical water ratios contributing to the swollen or puffy look you'd give anything to be rid of.

It is not always easy to detect sine the body has the capacity to absorb plenty of excess water, but there are ways to spot it if you know what to look out for.

The first sign you have water retention is if you are used to seeing your abs or muscular vascularity, but are no longer able to and you haven't drastically altered your food intake or exercise level.

Another sign, or actual test you can conduct on yourself, involves gently pressing an area of skin with your finger for about five seconds. An indent that remains after you remove the pressure of your fingers indicates water retention. Additionally, stretched and shiny skin covering swollen areas and rapid weight gain over a short period of time without an extreme excess of calories is another indicator.

Other symptoms that are telling and indicate you will benefit from this program include swollen ankles, feet and legs, especially at the end of a long day of standing or sitting, your rings feeling tighter than they used to be, your shoe size increasing after you've gone through puberty, or experiencing premenstrual bloating.

Gravity tends to pull water to the lower extremities, causing them to become bigger than normal. Also, look for puffiness of your arms, hands, face and around your eyes, as these are also clues about the water being stored in your body.

The common terminology used in these worlds is cutting water weight, and while it takes a great strength of will to accomplish double digit losses in single digit day spans, it is definitely possible.

CHAPTER 1

DISCLAIMERS AND PRECAUTIONS

Who And What This Book Is For

Believe it or not, I have wanted to write this book for a very long time and I have spent almost a year putting this together. The reasons are simple – it's a topic I am fascinated with and surprisingly, there is no other book dedicated solely to fast and safe water weight loss on the market. Given the large number of people, the professional and layperson alike, attempting to manipulate water weight for one reason or another, this book is sorely needed in the market.

Although I am a huge proponent of allocating enough time to lose weight slowly and steadily so that you are less likely to get into a pattern of yo-yo dieting, I live in the real world and happen to be a realist; so to anyone who might claim this book irresponsible, I think it's quite the opposite.

The reality is people procrastinate and look for shortcuts to lose weight all the time or simply need an extra boost to bolster them out of a plateau or add on top of their steady progress. It is a bonafide fact that hundreds of thousands of laypeople and weight-class based athletes will attempt to lose weight rapidly regardless of this book. Therefore, I'm simply trying to provide safer guidelines.

I do not want to encourage casual sex among high school students, either, but I recognize that the message to just say no and abstain doesn't work and results in unintended pregnancies, etc. I would rather have an open discussion and offer education to those who will do it regardless, which is the vast majority.

When it comes to the needs and wants of the vast majority, the word is already out - water weight is the easiest variable in weight loss to tackle and delivers the near instant results people seek. Plus, we can all agree that most people are constantly battling with a few extra pounds they would rather not have, so a relatively painless and quick solution to their problem will always be tempting to try. To illustrate my point, can you think of anyone you know who would say no to losing a quick five pounds from their frame?

Undoubtedly, there are still people who will argue that it is irresponsible to give step-by-step instructions on how to alter water retention because it is seen as a short cut or cop out to losing weight the so-called proper way. As the author of *"The Thigh Gap Hack"*, I'm pretty used to self-righteous critics and detractors who have nothing better in life to do than to judge what everyone else chooses to do with their bodies and turn their noses up at anyone who does things remotely different than what they narrow-mindedly deem right.

Luckily, I realize every person and scenario is not the same and therefore can only share what I know in hopes that it will be used for good rather than taken to the extreme and abused.

You see, I know for a fact that for some folks, quick weight loss may spark confidence and stick-with-it-ness towards a long-term, balanced diet and exercise program. On the other hand, other scenarios must be taken into context as they specifically call for last minute results and have nothing to do with a person's willpower or procrastinating proclivities.

Let's face it, every once in a while a special occasion comes before we are quite ready for it. You could have dieted and exercised for months only to come up just a few pound shy of your goal weight on the day of the event. Who is anyone to say whether or not doing my program to push yourself towards the finish line is morally or ethically wrong or encouraging bad habits?

Should a professional model who may have gained five pounds on vacation and returns home to find he/she has to unexpectedly get back to comp card measurements for a career defining gig be precluded from using these techniques when they are safe options that she can utilize to help her meet her goal?

Then there are instances where it is in the best interest for people to lose as little fat as possible while still shedding weight. For instance, fighters and power lifters specifically want to only shed enough water weight to get into a lower weight class when weighed a few hours before their fight, so that later on they can be back to their fuller, hydrated butt kicking bodies and have the upper hand over their much smaller, in body fat and muscles, competitor.

The point is everyone has his or her own reason to want to focus on overall weight and water loss versus fat loss, and it is not my job to judge or condemn your reasons for wanting this information. I only ask that you follow the instructions that I set out to the letter because if you are going to do this, you should do it properly to pose minimal risk to your health.

Remarkably, I personally know and have observed many professional athletes or fitness pros go about dropping water weight in the most inane and dangerous ways possible. Of course, it is worth noting that plenty of every day people, who are not competing in any type of sport or trying to get cast in a production - where being slender or meeting a certain weight benchmark is a part of the job description - also strive to lose weight fast by dropping water weight using dumb and potentially harmful strategies as well.

Precautions

I am sure everyone on this planet can sympathize with needing to drop a few pounds fast for a special event like a wedding, reunion, vacation, party, etc. We are all human and no one, not even the ridiculously fit bikini model with fifteen percent body fat can or will maintain her peak condition year round. That is why it's called your peak condition.

The dictionary defines peak of or relating to a period of highest use or demand. In other words, it's a high point surrounded by two lower points. Therefore, any shape you can stay in all year round is not your peak and when striving towards that high point it helps to have numerous options at your disposal.

When you can implement fat cutting techniques here, water cutting techniques there, and motivational techniques when necessary, it all adds up. This is the missing piece of the puzzle that unfortunately has been ignored for far too long.

That being said, it can be extremely dangerous to tackle significant water weight loss haphazardly. Some of the possible side effects are dehydration, fatigue, nausea and dizziness, electrolyte abnormalities, dependence, and heart or colon damage in the long term, so you don't want to attempt drastic weight loss without taking the necessary precautions and having a plan.

I will talk in more detail about all of the dangers in a little bit, but suffice to say the purpose of this book is to lay out a safe and effective way to lose water weight for professional athletes or sports competitors, fitness pros, models and lay people alike, because no one should undertake quick weight loss like the one promised in this title unless they have done their research and know exactly what they are doing or are under the care and guidance of a professional.

What This Book is Not

You now know what this book is and who it is for, but to be crystal clear, what this book is *not* is a long-term solution to weight or fat loss. First, because as we have already discussed the techniques outlined in the plans are for water loss, and not fat loss. There is a marked difference.

Second, the tactics and protocols I am about to divulge are intense! In fact, they are so intense that I have only included protocols that specifically are to be done in the short term – some tactics should only be used for up to two weeks at a time while others only once every few months. Unlike my other books, *"The Thigh Gap Hack"* and *"Bye-Bye Thunder Thighs"*, you won't find me advocating these plans as long-term lifestyle changes.

Third and lastly, unlike fat loss, which requires eating in an excess of 3500 calories to put back on one pound that is lost (one pound of fat equals 3500 calories), simply eating a few starchy tubers or fruit will signal your body to start holding on to that water in a matter of hours.

Do not get me wrong, after initially losing water weight it is entirely possible for you to minimize the amount of water your body retains in the future by eating smart long term, but don't expect every single ounce of it to stay off even with careful dieting/exercise. That time of the month, and one or a few days of backsliding and letting loose just a little bit could leave you frustrated and disappointed if your expectations are not realistic.

The typical rules that you might hear at the end of a strong weight loss product being advertised on the radio or television also apply. If you are high-risk, elderly, pregnant, nursing, or have any chronic diseases or other serious medical issue, this plan might not be for you. Why? Again, because you might seriously injure or harm yourself if you have other pre-existing conditions and overtax your body.

To summarize, if you realize the limitations, accept them and have realistic expectations, are otherwise a healthy individual and would like to drop a bunch of water weight fast for a special occasion, whether it be to fit into a wedding dress or one-up the competition, you have the green light to proceed reading.

If you would like a more balanced, long term diet and exercise plan that will promise definite fat loss along, where water weight will also diminish – albeit slowly, I encourage you to check out one of my best selling books, *The Thigh Gap Hack* or *Bye-Bye Thunder Thighs*. Also feel free to delve into the plethora of helpful free articles and resources on my blog, http://www.thighgaphack.com.

CHAPTER 2

HOW WATER WEIGHT WORKS

How it Works

In the grand scheme of things how much you weigh probably won't matter so much to you unless your goal is to hit a certain number on the scale for a competition, and then it matters a great deal. For the rest of you, what you are most likely concerned about is how you actually look and how your clothes fit.

I have got good news for everyone; *'How to Lose Water Weight'* has got you covered on all fronts. Think about the size and appearance of a filled water balloon versus an empty deflated balloon and you can imagine the remarkable difference in weight and appearance to be had by reducing the amount of water your body currently stores.

To put things into perspective, a gallon of water weighs 8 pounds and a pint of water (16 ounces) weighs 1 pound. Yes, it is quite amazing how much the small compound of $H20$ can weight. That being said, let's go over the way water weight actually works. We will begin with a pretty easy to grasp concept as it pertains to weight and its relation to water retention.

Weight is defined as a body's relative mass or the quantity of matter contained by it, giving rise to a downward force or the heaviness of a person or thing. At the risk of stating the obvious, we measure the weight of something with scales.

However, when it comes to the body's weight, scales measure not just body fat and muscle, but also bone, organs (like your lungs, heart and liver), bodily fluids, waste inside your digestive system you haven't yet eliminated, and glycogen (the form of carbohydrate your body uses as back up fuel, which is stored with water).

Water weight is the generic term for the weight on your body solely due to water. We already know the human body is mostly made up of water; that includes both inside and outside our body's cells. For instance blood is more than 80% water, bones are 50% water, fat is 10% - 30% water, and muscle is 75% water.

Whereas water weight encompasses all the weight on your body due to water, water retention signifies an abnormal accumulation of fluid within the cavity or tissues of the body and in the circulatory system. That excessive water plays a significant role in your total weight and is also classified as water weight since it is water that contributes to your weight.

Another way to put this is that all water retention counts as body water, but not all of your body water is due to water retention. Got it? Good.

The water weight we will tackle and strive to decrease is the normal levels of water in and outside the body's cells as well as the abnormal levels of water in the circulatory system, cavities, and below the skin as a result of water retention.

Weight loss in a short period of time, like a day or so, will mainly consist of water outside of the cells. This is because exercise physiologists tell us you cannot lose fat and muscles, which contains water inside the cells, unless you are in a calorie deficit or the calories in, calories out theory.

Undoubtedly you've heard the calories in, calories out theory before, but just in case you are not familiar, this paradigm states that in order to experience weight loss, you must reduce the amount of calories ingested or absorbed and/or increase the amount of energy expended (via exercise, non-exercise activity, cold thermogenesis, etc.).

Longer weight loss endeavors - over a few weeks or a month - will include water weight loss as a result of your fat cells being reduced, possibly some muscle loss, as well as from glycogen, bodily fluids and waste being released. Just as with fat, muscle loss takes some time. Decreasing protein and using fewer weights when working out, since they both result in water retention, and eating at a deficit all contribute to muscle mass loss. This works out swimmingly well for people who want to lose overdeveloped bulky muscles.

With one-day to one-week timelines, glycogen, bodily fluids and waste inside your digestive system are what you should be specifically targeting. These variables are constantly fluctuating and by focusing on diet/nutrition and other methodologies we can quickly and drastically alter these factors so that they result in you weighing a lot less on the scale.

Two-week timelines on the other hand, will include water weight from true fat loss and perhaps some slight muscle loss. Just so we are clear, you will not be able to lose water from your organs, or bones on this or any other weight loss plan, nor should you have to since we want these parts of us to be fully functioning as designed.

CHAPTER 3

THE MAJOR PLAYERS

Far Reaching VS Low Hanging Fruit

Now that we know how body water and water retention works and the overall sources of water weight loss, let's delve deeper into the details and divide them into two categories – the low hanging fruit (glycogen, bodily fluid, and waste) and the far-reaching fruit (fat and muscles).

Bear in mind that despite these categories, there are only four ways to actually get the water out of your body - urine, sweat, feces, and respiration, or the air you exhale. Therefore, when we talk about losing water weight by eliminating fat and muscle, that water will actually exit the body as one of those four ways (waste).

WASTE

Every time you eat or drink you temporarily put on the weight of that item in the short term. For example, if you were to weigh yourself, eat a pound of chicken and vegetables, and then step back on the scale immediately afterwards, your weight will increase by one pound. It is no different than putting a bunch of rocks in your pocket.

This is why in my other books I stress that obsessing over the scale and weighing yourself every day is not a good idea. Weight alone is simply not the best barometer of fat loss. This is also the reason behind the recommendation to weigh yourself at the same time of day every time (e.g. first thing in the morning before eating or drinking) if you want to get an accurate idea of your actual progress.

The key to not gaining any weight ultimately from the one-pound of food in the example above is to excrete from your body at least one-pound.

Logically, the question is, if we gain weight whenever we eat or drink, do we lose said weight whenever we use the restroom? Not quite – we will lose weight when we use the rest room but not all of it will come from your last meal, which is attested by the fact that many of us have compacted waste in the colon or sitting around in our body weighing in the double digits (up to thirty pounds, with bigger people carrying more).

Besides, if we did lose all the weight of the foods we consumed whenever we used the restroom, we'd never have to worry about putting on weight. Of course, there's no denying that we do. So what exactly happens and how does food and waste affect your weight in the longer run?

Some hours after you eat something, your body will convert some of the food to energy to operate your body. Some of it will be discarded as waste, and any energy excess will be stored for later use by the body as fat. The ratios of energy used, amount of waste, and amount stored for later will depend on your current energy needs and how exactly your particular body converts the particular food you ate.

It is important to note for some given food your body may be able to extract a very high percentage of the energy in that food, while the next person may only be able to get a very small amount of energy out of it.

How many hours it takes you to process food depends on how much you ate, what you ate, and how fast your body processes that food. Each person is likely to process the same food at a different rate. Your body also processes different foods at different rates.

The rough timeline though from the sequence of ingestion, digestion, and egestion spans twelve hours on average, and by the time the residual waste of food is passed out, some parts, the useable ones, have all been put to use for energy expenditure, as heat generation, or placed into storage, as either glycogen (from carbohydrate), or fat.

Our goal then is to get as much as we can of the foods we consume and digest passed out as waste (the low hanging fruit) – and we will cover precisely how to achieve that in the upcoming sections. Additionally, our goal is to eliminate any current waste from your system that is currently contributing to your weight.

BODILY FLUID

Tackling body fluids is the next easiest way to eliminate water weight. Body fluids are defined as liquids originating from inside the bodies of living humans. They include fluids that are excreted or secreted from the body. While the list of our bodily fluids is long, the two types that pertain to our objectives are urine and perspiration or sweat.

The average person eliminates about 1 liter a day through perspiration. Now that's a lot of weight lost without much effort. Imagine what could be achieved if you purposefully began to sweat more. The obvious answer is you'd lose even more weight.

The school of thought on sweating to lose weight is a mixed bag. Some people are big believers in it and others criticize the practice for not having very lasting results and/or putting people who take it to the extreme at a serious risk of injury.

My response to those who think it too potentially dangerous to manipulate is that technically, anything done to an extreme for too long can harm you. Drinking too much water could lead to a condition known as water intoxication, which is when a person drinks so much water that the other nutrients in the body become diluted to the point that they can no longer do their jobs. Yet you rightfully won't hear people warning you to stay away from water at all costs.

The truth of the matter is sweating is indeed an effective and easy way to drop weight, hence its inclusion in the low hanging fruit category. Also contrary to popular opinion, you can see the effects of weight loss from sweating for longer than a few minutes or your next trip to the water fountain.

Some people have reported weight loss from sweating that has lasted up to a few weeks, and given many of the protocols I will recommend can be done in the comfort of your own home, you can mitigate water retention for an even longer period by sweating it out regularly (once or twice a month).

As for urine, it's pretty easy to understand how urinating more will lead to the loss of water weight. If you're anything like the average person, you are currently already eliminating about 1.2 liters of water in urine each day. But unlike popular opinion, urine is more complex than just that drink you had a few hours ago.

Simply abstaining from drinking any water won't exactly get you to avoid weight gain, just as drinking more water won't guarantee the flood gates will be released. That is because when water is restricted without a strategic plan, the body compensates by reducing the amount of urine excreted. Similarly, sometimes gulping down lots of water will simply result in the body retaining it if you haven't created the proper environment for that water to be released.

That is not to say we won't be utilizing either of these techniques – in fact, we most surely will. There are just unique and precise conditions under which both approaches will work, which we'll go over later. I say all of that to stress there must be a method to the madness to get your desired results.

In a nutshell, the body produces urine as a way to get rid of waste and extra water it does not need as a result of digestion and metabolism. The key players in this scenario are the kidneys, which filters waste from the blood and produce urine to get rid of it.

Therefore, to lose water weight with urine, you can either stimulate the kidney, find a way to help the body metabolize faster, get your body to let go of the water it retains due to various factors (which we will discuss in the next chapter) or target glycogen, fat and muscle loss as it will be expelled in the form of urine.

GLYCOGEN

Your body stores energy in one of two ways, either as fat and glycogen. Whereas the amount of fat stores varies from person to person, your body can only store so much energy as glycogen. Just in case you're bewildered by the statement above and wondering about where the nutrients, protein, dietary fat and carbohydrates fits in the puzzle, I'll explain carbohydrates here and the other two very shortly.

First, in order to understand glycogen we have to start with glucose. Glucose is a simple sugar that provides the body with its primary source of energy. This type of sugar comes from digesting carbohydrates into a chemical that the body can easily convert to energy. Glycogen is the main way the body stores glucose for later use and is the typically the first to be depleted in the earliest phases of any diet.

A good way to think of glycogen is as a fuel tank full of stored carbohydrates. The name carbo*hydrate*, which means "watered carbon" or carbon with attached water molecules, hints at the fact glycogen requires water to be stored. It is stored in the liver, muscles, and fat cells in hydrated form (three to four parts water) associated with potassium.

In other words, there are, on average, four calories per gram of carbohydrate and for every gram of carbohydrate we eat; we store 3 grams of water. Feel free to latch on to this point, because it's critical. It's already normal fare to experience glycogen and water weight shifts of up to two pounds per day in either direction (gain or loss) even with no changes in your calorie intake or activity level. If you're eating a lot of carbohydrates, you're gaining and storing a lot of water, and if you cut out carbohydrates or deplete your carbohydrate stores, the water weight follows by taking a dip.

But wait, there's more. The energy deficit required to reduce weight with glycogen as fuel at 1800 kcal per pound is far less than fat at 3500 kcal per pound, due to the difference in every contribution of fat versus carbohydrate, and the large amount of water associated with storage glycogen. To put this fact into perspective, you would need to eat 3500 calories less per week versus 1800 calories less per week to lose one pound of weight.

This is one of the reasons people on The Atkins Diet, or any other low carb / ketogenic diet, will experience rapid weight loss at the start of their diet and why frequent urination is one of the side effects of these types of diets.

The brain receives a signal that the body is not getting the same calories and food and sends impulses to activate the storehouse of energy to compensate. The body utilizes the energy reserves, which stores glycogen in your liver and muscles, and leads to the production of energy in the form of ATP molecules and water.

Breaking down glycogen releases a lot of water. As your carb intake and glycogen stores drop, your kidneys will start dumping the excess water. In addition, as your circulating insulin levels drop, your kidneys start excreting excess sodium, which will also cause more frequent urination.

FAT

It is general knowledge that if you lose adipose tissue, or body fat, you lose weight (the good and more long-lasting kind) on the scale, but did you know that sometimes you will fail to lose the full amount of weight that you theoretically should, if you subscribe to the calories in/ calories out theory, because of our good friend, water?

Before I expound on the above, I want you to have a full picture of the way fat is digested and stored in the body, and the overall workings of fat as we have done for carbohydrates, glucose and glycogen above.

The digestion of dietary fat begins in the mouth, where food is first broken down into smaller components, mixed with lingual lipase found in your saliva, and swallowed. Digestion then continues in the stomach, but most fat digestion takes place in the small intestine.

In the small intestine, bile stored in the gall bladder is released and emulsifies the fats into smaller droplets that are absorbed into the blood stream. Any extra fatty acids are stored as adipose tissue, better known as body fat.

One thing that needs to be clarified is if you are eating in a deficit, you will indeed lose fat along with water weight. However, it is still possible to lose water weight without losing fat if you are not eating at a deficit, e.g. eating at maintenance. To further complicate things, you can still continue to lose weight no matter how much water weight you are carrying, but we are getting ahead of ourselves.

To see drastic results on short term plans where you only have a mere twenty four hours, you can create a calorie deficit but even if you fast all day, it won't be enough to burn significant fat that will lead to considerable weight loss on the scale. This is why we primarily focus on manipulating water weight in a time crunch.

On longer plans, you can accumulate enough of a calorie deficit to result in decent fat loss of five to ten pounds. This is where we circle back to the opening statement that I promised I would expound upon. Everything can be on point but fat loss

31

still may not be readily apparent on the scale because water is said to fill the fat cells as triaglycerol (how fat is stored inside of the fat cell) decreases or is released into the bloodstream as free fatty acids.

While science isn't conclusive on the matter, the widely held theory is that as fat is burned through dieting and a calorie deficit and removed from the cell, water is used to keep the cell structurally sound resulting in the fat loss being obscured or hidden to the naked eye and our weight loss detection devices.

If that sounds really depressing, I promise it gets better. At a certain trigger point one of three things happen: (1) The cell cannibalizes the cell membrane and shrinks, (2) the cell becomes similar to a phagocyte, meaning it drops volume but retains surface area, or (3) the cell dies decreasing the number of adipose cells – although some studies assert that the body simply replenishes those cells, albeit with a lowered volume, and that we maintain the same number of cells in adulthood.

Other evidence supporting the above is a phenomenon known as "dieter's edema", which is where after a while of cutting calories the body retains a large amount of water. One of the effects observed is a shift in the water content of the fat cells. Normally water would represent 10~14% of the fat cell volume but can be far more during this dieter's edema phenomena.

Our objective is to speed the process along of emptying out the water from the fat cell while you lose fat, or try to prevent it in the first place, so that fat loss becomes apparent sooner.

There is nothing quite as frustrating eating and exercising in a manner that should result in weight loss, but seeing a stall on the scale and in the mirror so I know you can't wait to learn how to thwart one of mother nature's cruelest tricks. As such, we'll discuss our best defenses, re-feeds, intermittent fasting, and full-blown fasts in the upcoming chapters.

PROTEIN / MUSCLES

Last, but not least in the weight loss culprit list is Protein. Protein can actually be manipulated in more than one way when it comes to weight loss.

First, diminished protein intake coupled with a low calorie diet can and will result in muscle loss, which we have already covered is made up of 75% water. So when you lose muscle, you lose water and subsequently more weight. This is only relevant for people (mostly women) who would prefer to lose overdeveloped muscles. Secondly, protein is one of nutrients that must be used when you need to diminish carbs and deplete your glycogen stores.

At face value, it might seem like I've made completely conflicting statements – as in one sentence you have the recommendation to diminish protein and the other to increase protein. As usual, it's all under the context of how much time you have to get the job done and overall body desires.

First, let's talk about protein as a nutrient and the substitution of carbs to lose water weight. We already know that carbs, which contributes mostly to your glycogen stores, results in the body holding on to a lot of water. Therefore, it would make sense to reduce the amount of carbs you eat if you need to lose water weight fast.

However, when you cut out a large chunk of one nutrient from your diet, you have to compensate elsewhere or else you might find yourself on a very low calorie diet. Since very low calorie isn't necessary to lose water weight in the extremely short term (a full day of fasting still wouldn't be enough for most people to burn a pound of fat) the calories that you are no longer consuming in carbs can be made up in protein.

The reason we use protein to do the job is because whereas fat has nine calories per gram, protein only contains four. Protein also takes longer to digest, thus making you feel satisfied longer. Finally, it's hard to over eat protein, which is why you don't see too many people binging on fish or grilled chicken.

It's worth pointing out here that the above isn't a green light to surpass or even replace the amount of carb calories with protein calories down to the number. That's because too much protein will lead to fat gain. To further explain, when you eat foods containing protein, the protein is broken down into building blocks known as peptides, and then further broken down into amino acids. The amino acids are absorbed through the small intestine's lining and enter the blood stream.

From there, some is used to build the body's protein stores. Excess amino acids is broken down and converted into sugars or fatty acids (fat/weight gain), not used to build muscle as commonly thought. To be extra clear, protein does help to build muscle, but only under the condition that you have torn the muscles (by working them out intensely - which we cover in the exercise chapter).

Any excess protein after the muscles have been filled, or excess protein with no muscle to repair either goes to waste or is stored as fat. Now you can understand why it's ridiculous for people trying to lose weight to guzzle protein shakes, typically loaded in protein and calories, for breakfast, dinner or lunch without the intention of breaking a sweat.

The second way protein plays a role in weight loss is its relation to muscle. When you have been eating at a large calorie deficit for a few weeks in an attempt to lose considerable weight, whether you tear those muscles or not, if you do not consume enough protein you are bound to some muscle.

We are not talking copious amounts here, but definitely enough to affect your overall weight and your water weight levels because as we know, when you lose some of your muscles you also lose some of the water that gets stored inside of those fibers.

I will lay out the guidelines for how much protein is not enough, and if you should be striving to tear those muscles or not during your workout when attempting a big cut via a large calorie deficit later on.

CHAPTER 4

WATER RETENTION CAUSES

Why the Body Retains Water

The body and internal organs are made up of water because water is a necessary medium for nearly all of the reactions that are involved in the function of life. Without it, the body's cells could not work properly; they would soon fail and effectively die, resulting in disease, injury to and death of the whole organism.

That being said, there are many reasons our bodies retain or store more water than normal and ultimately, our aim is to battle this aspect of water retention versus the essential levels of water. The water retention that you want to target to look leaner is called subcutaneous fluid. This is fluid that is located under your skin and is caused by water molecules bonding onto to sodium ions.

Take note that while we want to reduce your body fluid to aid in weight loss, water retention could result in various health problems, such as kidney disorders and joint pain. Acute water retention can even result in heart problems.

When deciding what to include and omit, I settled on including a separate chapter to the how and why of water retention instead of briefly skimming or listing the reasons because if you can understand the cause and effect, you become aware of opportunities to change your behavior. Brace yourself though, because the list is long.

For instance, some common causes of water retention include hot weather, obesity, high salt diet, blood clots, vascular problems, sitting or standing for a long time, allergies, insect bites, infection, hormonal changes during menstruation and pregnancy, high or low blood pressure and as a side effect to some medications. However, serious medical conditions such as congestive heart failure, liver cirrhosis, kidney damage, damaged veins and an inadequate lymphatic system may also lead to accumulation of water in the tissues.

Salt / Sodium

Believe it or not, salt does not have any calories so it doesn't cause your body to store or gain fat directly. However, it is one of the most common culprits for temporary water weight gain and does have an indirect link to fat/weight gain. The reason is that high levels of salt in our diets usually come from calorie dense, fiber poor, processed foods.

Our bodies rely on electrolytes, most significantly sodium and potassium, to carry the electrical impulses that control our bodily functions. In order for our bodies to function properly, it is important that the concentration of electrolytes in our bodies remain constant.

A high concentration of electrolytes in our blood triggers our thirst mechanism, causing us to consume adequate amounts of water to return to the proper concentration of electrolytes. When we consume an adequate amount of water, our kidneys are able to keep the concentration of electrolytes in our blood constant by increasing or decreasing the amount of water we retain.

However, the water moves beyond our bloodstream. Through the process of osmosis, water flows from a lower salinity environment to a higher one in an attempt to balance the levels of salinity. After we consume large amounts of salt, it is the water moving from our bloodstream into our skin that gives us water retention. Then, when we consume lesser amounts of salt, the same process works in reverse to remove the excess water from our bodies.

While the recommended daily intake of sodium is 1500mg, for most people consumer on average 2500+ mg. Now just because 1500 mg is the recommended average doesn't mean it's a healthy amount. My book, *Bye-Bye Thunder Thighs,* goes into details on how the food pyramid, upheld as a widely lauded template everyone should follow, was corrupted by backroom dealings with the food industry giants in more detail.

In reality, 500 mg a day is sufficient enough and will result in less water retention as well as lowered blood pressure. Keep in mind that there is sodium in everything - even fruits and vegetables, so while it is impossible to have a 0 sodium diet, it is possible to have a 0-added-sodium-diet and strive towards a lower sodium diet overall.

Climate / Hot Weather

Significant changes in body weight due to climate usually take the form of weight gained rather than weight lost, especially once the body has become acclimated to high levels of activity in the heat. This might seem counterintuitive, since we tend to sweat more in warm weather, but while our complex body seems to do backwards and unexpected things from time to time; there is a method to its madness.

When it's hot and humid outside, body weight can go up by several pounds due to increased body water through fluid-conserving hormones such as aldosterone. Aldosterone allows the kidney to retain more fluid and reduces the amount of salt in sweat, leading to even more water retention.

Additionally, while we do sweat in heat increased temperatures and water in the air have the effect of rendering the body's cooling mechanism, sweating, useless. Yes, humid weather will increase the sweating rate, but in high humidity, sweat typically drips off the body rather than evaporating, thus providing no cooling effect. As a result, you stay hot. The hotter you are, the more water you'll retain.

Another way weather effects water retention is, as the climate changes the body adapts via a process known as heat acclimatization in order to reduce the negative effects of heat stress. After a few days of heat acclimatization, sweating starts sooner and takes place at higher rates, improving evaporative cooling and reducing body heat storage and skin temperature.

Thus, after heat acclimatization, fluid requirements will be higher due to increased sweating. Heat acclimatization also improves fluid balance by better matching thirst to water needs, increasing the blood volume and increasing total body water.

Finally, hotter temperatures and intense exercise increase sweating rates and, as a result, water requirements. If we don't comply we are left dehydrated, which prompts the body to hold on to as much water as possible.

Damaged Veins

Water retention is sometimes caused by damage to or pressure within veins that causes them to leak fluid — blood plasma that is mostly water — into nearby tissue.

Lymphatic System

The lymphatic system is part of the circulatory system, comprising a network of lymphatic vessels that carry a clear fluid called lymph directionally towards the heart. It acts like an "overflow" and can return a lot of excess fluid back to the bloodstream, but can be overwhelmed.

If there is simply too much fluid, or if the lymphatic system is congested, then the fluid will remain in the tissues and/or leak into the surrounding tissue causing swellings in legs, ankles, feet, abdomen or any other part of the body.

Allergies

When an inflammation is present in the body, histamine is released. Histamine causes the gaps between the cells of the capillary walls to widen, making them more leaky. The aim is to make it easier for infection-fighting white cells to quickly get to the site of an inflammation (infection). However, if the inflammation persists for a long time, water retention can become chronic (long-term).

The body naturally manufactures histamine and releases it in the presence of allergens. Allergens can be insect bites, pollen, or any foreign compound that the body develops a reaction to. The allergen in question can be very specific to the individual. Histamine causes water retention by causing capillaries to dilate and allowing them to leak fluid. This normally is beneficial, because it releases white blood cells and fluid to injured or infected tissue.

Hormonal Changes

A complex system of hormones and prostaglandins (hormone-like substances) is used by the human body to regulate water levels so that excess water intake one day can be resolved by the kidneys quickly excreting the excess urine, while a lack of fluids on another day may result in much less urination that usual.

Certain hormones and medications, such as insulin, cortisone, and estrogen, can also affect how your body regulates its sodium levels and lead to water weight.

Finally, during menstruation and pregnancy there can be hormone imbalances, as well as some nutritional factors that will lead to water retention. With pregnancy, hormones encourage the body to hold onto excess fluid, while women on the pill will see water retention because oral contraceptives that include oestrogen can trigger it.

Kidney Damage

Our kidneys carry out the complex system of filtration in our bodies - excess waste and fluid material are removed from the blood and excreted from the body. Our kidneys get their blood and oxygen supply from the renal arteries, which are branches of the abdominal aorta (another artery). When it enters the kidneys, blood goes through smaller and smaller blood vessels - the smallest ones being the glomeruli (tiny capillary blood vessels which are arranged in tufts).

Kidney damage is a rapid (days to weeks) decline in the kidneys' ability to filter metabolic waste products from the blood. Causes include disorders that decrease blood flow to the kidneys, that damage the kidneys themselves, or that block drainage of urine from the kidneys.

In most cases our kidneys are able to eliminate all waste materials that our body produces. However, if the blood flow to the kidneys is affected, or the tubules or glomeruli are not working properly because of damage or disease, or if urine outflow is obstructed, problems can occur. Including kidney failure - then waste material, including fluids, cannot be eliminated (shed) from the body properly, resulting in fluid retention.

Liver Damage

The liver is the largest organ in the body and one of the most essential. It may be injured by a single event, as in acute (new, short-term) hepatitis; by regular injury over months or years, as in biliary tract blockage or chronic hepatitis; or by continuous injury, as in daily alcohol abuse.

Damage to the normal liver tissue that keeps this important organ from working as it should is called Cirrhosis. If the damage is not stopped, the liver gradually loses its ability to carry out its normal functions. Severe cirrhosis that triggers liver failure causes fluid retention by putting you at risk for infections and high pressures force fluid out of your blood vessels into your liver, pooling it in your abdomen, causing swelling and dehydration.

Additionally, as fluid pools in your abdomen, your kidneys will try to hold onto more water, because they think your body is dehydrated. The excess fluid collects in your lungs, legs and abdomen.

Infection

Have you ever noticed that whenever you get an infection, that area of your body swells or puffs up? This is a telltale sign that you have water retention on your hands, figuratively and sometimes literally.

The swelling is caused by an accumulation of fluid in tissues as your macrophages (guard cells that guard every border region of the boy) order the blood vessels to release water into the battlefield so fighting your infection become easier. Therefore the swelling is is in fact your body's attempt to push foreign material out.

Heart Failure

Normal pressure within blood vessels is partly maintained by the pumping force of the heart. However, if the heart starts to fail (congestive heart failure), the body compensates in various ways. It starts to retain fluid and increase the volume of blood.

There will be congestion of the veins, fluid build up in the lungs, and other parts of the body, enlargement of the liver, a change in blood pressure (this pressure backs up in the heart), which often results in serious water retention, typically manifested as swelling (oedema) in the legs and feet.

Obesity

Severe obesity can result in insidious fluid retention, which can be easily overlooked by the gradual and insidious accumulation of fluid until large volumes of fluid have accumulated.

In severe obesity there can be multiple contributors to the oedema. Hypertension, diabetes, sleep disordered breathing, 'obesity-related asthma', non-alcoholic fatty liver, focal-segmental glomerulo-sclerosis, low physical fitness levels, thromboembolic disease, lymphoedema, and vitamin deficiencies are all common.

Obesity also potentiates the sympathetic activation seen in heart failure leading to renin-angiotensin-aldosterone axis activation, resulting in further salt and fluid accumulation. Additionally, people who are bedridden, confined to wheelchairs, or just plain couch potatoes can experience water retention due to a lack of circulation in their bloodstreams that would otherwise occur during mobile activity.

Scan through the other causes of fluid retention in this chapter and you will see how obesity impacts all of the relevant areas of the body that contribute towards water retention.

Vascular Problems

Blood clots. of, relating to, affecting, or consisting of a vessel or vessels, especially those that carry blood. The result of our retaining more or less water in our bloodstream can also affect our blood pressure.

Venous insufficiency is a common problem caused by weakened valves in the veins of the legs. This makes it more difficult for the veins to pump blood back to the heart, and leads to varicose veins and build up of fluid.

Sitting or Standing for Long Times

Sitting or standing for long periods of time leads to water retention in the ankles because blood pools or builds up in the lower extremities, such as the legs.

Too Little or Too Much Water

Not drinking enough fluids can lead to water retention as your body's attempt to counter dehydration (Other causes of dehydration include drinking lots of alcohol or too many caffeinated drinks). What happens is if you ingest enough water, the kidneys do not try and retain water by cutting back on elimination.

On the flip side of the coin, as previously noted too much water isn't the answer. A lot of people blindly strive to follow the advice to drink eight or more 8-ounce classes of water a day – and if they're not meeting the requirement at least feel guilty about it.

The truth is under extreme conditions when you are drinking more than 12 liters in twenty-four hours or exercising heavily — to disrupt the body's osmotic balance by diluting and flushing too much sodium, an electrolyte that helps balance the pressure of fluids inside and outside of cells. That means cells bloat from the influx and may even burst. Extreme overconsumption of water can also strain the kidneys and, if drunk with meals, interfere with proper digestion.

Additionally consuming lots of water alongside high intensity workouts and heavy lifting can lead to bloating as the muscles store excess water to help with the repair process.

CHAPTER 5

WHAT TO EXPECT

It may seem unnecessary to those of you who want to get down to brass tacks, but everything we have covered up until now has been crucial. I don't just want you to take my word for how and why this stuff works, but to understand for yourself how and why following the plan will be beneficial to your goals of losing water weight.

Hopefully, after you've set down the book and gone through your initial water weight journey you will be conscientious of things you need to continue doing as well as avoid doing because you will have a deeper understanding of the implications.

Now that you have a very clear idea of the physiological concepts (understanding the science of the function of the living systems) and logic behind how water works in the body, we're inching closer yet to the meat and potatoes portion of this book.

In the subtitle of this book, I have already revealed the results that are possible in terms of how much water weight you can lose in how much time and how differently your body can look, but it doesn't end there because you aren't going to finish reading this book and magically lose the weight. You will have to actually apply the plan I lay out and thus, I want to adequately prepare you for what lies ahead.

Right off the bat, if you do not think you'll be able to dedicate yourself to the rigors of the diet, it's okay. Maybe you're going through an already stressful period in your life or your mental or physical health is not where it needs to be to see the plan through. If that's the case, don't feel an iota of guilt about putting this book down and coming back to it when you're ready to follow the instructions to a tee.

The first thing I want you to know is that weight loss is not linear, it happens in stops and starts. The reason is because every body is unique, operates under different variables, and therefore will be a bit unpredictable or unruly. It makes sense then that you will need to exercise patience while sticking to the plan until your body decides to catch up and fall in line with your goals.

It might seem counterintuitive to declare needing patience for a diet plan that promises incredible results super fast so let me explain. Have you ever heard the commonly referred to terminology, the whoosh effect?

The whoosh effect is a phenomenon where a person can be doing everything right in terms of diet and exercise for weeks with no results. Then, seemingly overnight, something

51

happens and the scale drops a bunch. Typically the rapid weight loss often follows a period of weight loss stall.

The point in telling you this is to prepare you for the fact that you might be doing a one week protocol and not see any results until day five or six when your body decides to play catch up all at once. Alternatively, you might see results on day two. There's no telling because we are all different and weight loss again is non-linear.

It's important to take this into consideration because of the psychological aspect of your immediate expectations not lining up to reality. For example, if after following the instructions to a tee and not seeing any payoff after four days, you might be confused, frustrated and tempted to give up early when success is right around the corner. Don't let that be the case – remember your whoosh effect will come if you are patient.

Another expectation you should have is to for your willpower to be extremely tested. Willpower is the ability to force yourself to do something that you don't particularly want to do in the moment or the ability to resist short-term temptations in order to meet long-term goals.

Think of it as a one shot thruster that burns out quickly, but if directed intelligently can provide the burst you need to overcome inertia and create momentum. Of course, this is much easier said than done but we'll get to how you can establish better willpower shortly.

For now, I can guarantee you that you will doubt yourself, fight hunger, thirst, a little birdie in your ear telling you to skip cardio, your friends and family, whose opinions you respect, regurgitating negative things they've heard regarding water weight manipulation – possibly not agreeing with the tactics you are using or telling you it's okay to veer from the hard parts in good natured attempt to be supportive.

It can be easy to buckle under the pressure, get distracted and give in to your emotions and inner limitations. To avoid this very common shortcoming, you need to establish a beachhead such that further progress can be made with far less effort than is required of the initial thrust.

Examples of beachheads would be buying a treadmill desk so you can be sure to get your cardio in while doing other mundane activities like watching television or surfing the internet, throwing out all junk food from your house and disposing of all juices so that you have no choice but to drink water, buying or pre-cooking a week's worth of low sodium, high fiber, low carb meals that will aid in getting rid of water retention, pre-setting the thermostat to automatically adjust to a higher temperature while you sleep, and/or altering your computer settings to block your favorite food blogs and social media sites (which tend to glorify food) to better adhere to your fasting period,

Doing all of the above is how you can use your temporary willpower to alter the territory around you in such a way that maintaining momentum won't be as hard as building it in the first place as you can implement all of the above in one day. Executing hard and fast in the beginning, while willpower is strong, is the key to your success.

It doesn't end there though. Additionally, you will need to have discipline to follow your diet and exercise routines. This is where a source of driving force to execute the plan originally set forth comes in handy.

Examples of sources of driving force include writing down in no uncertain terms your objective for starting this program in the first place. Be very detailed as possible, really delving deep in the whys and what it will mean to you to see the program through. Treat it as a cathartic exercise. Also include promises to yourself to give it your very best and to let nothing sidetrack you from your goal.

During times where it feels like you have lost sight of your goal, like when your willpower has waned and you are being tempted to indulge in a bowl of pasta or ice cream by a well-meaning friend, think back to or whip out your manifesto to yourself and read it.

If you have a picture of yourself at your goal weight, make sure that image is visible to you every day as a reminder of what it's all about and that you consult the image when your will power is put to the test. If you do not have such a picture of yourself, a picture of a model or celebrity whose body resembles reasonable your ultimate goal at the end of the program will suffice.

It is important to note that your fitspiration should reasonably look the way you hope to look after you've lost water weight on this program, and not of someone who has clearly been in the fitness game for eons, adhering to a crazy fitness and strict diet regiment for years.

Your results won't resemble their single digit body fat percentages, and you'll just feel dejected when you lose fifteen pounds but still look nothing like the (likely photoshopped) model you selected from Google images. This is why I would prefer the picture you use is of yourself at a more desirable weight. The reason for doing all of the above is to get something called emotional clarity.

Emotional clarity is when how we feel on the inside about what we are compelled to do is in alignment with what we intellectually believe we should do and it's the first step in developing discipline. The smaller your window of time and the greater your water weight loss goal, the more discipline you will need, albeit you will exercise that discipline for a shorter time.

In case some of you are wondering, there is a difference between will power and discipline. Self-discipline or self-control is a conscious act, while willpower is a general designation. To be clear, self-discipline is the conscious act of controlling one's mental facilities; it is purely psychological. It is not a course of actions leading to a certain goal or ideal, but the assertion of willpower over more base desires.

Self-discipline is to some extent a substitute for motivation, when one uses reason to determine the best course of action that opposes one's desires. Willpower is when successfully engaging in and maintaining for any length of time, the acts of self-discipline.

Therefore, the goal is to use willpower to immediately attack the environment and social obstacles that perpetuate the problem while making sure you have emotional clarity – a compelling reason to do the task you know you should do – whether it be your inspirational picture, letter to yourself with reminders of why losing the weight is so important to you, addressing your self worth fears, etc.

I happen to agree with the assertions that defense is the best offense and thusly, something you must gird yourself for is the end of the plan. You want to make sure you do not sink into developing issues with your eating habits or body image after the special occasion or event is over and done with.

It can be very flattering to hear people compliment you on the amount of weight you've lost and stroke your ego about how great you look. While some people can take those compliments and channel them into dedicating themselves to a lifestyle change that includes cutting out processed, junky, franken foods and fitting more movement or exercise in their days, it can also be all to easy to go in the complete opposite direction and do another round or three of the programs, which are not meant to be extended for a reason.

My hope is that if you realize upfront that at the end of this, it's a normal reaction to want to keep going for increased quick results but also know why you shouldn't, you will do a better job of talking yourself out of it.

To that point, what type of personality do you have? Are you meticulous and detail oriented? Great, you'll do very well with these programs. If you hate the idea of tracking your calories or fussing with details you can expect to either buckle down for a few days and find every tool possible to make the task easier or fail. I'm not mincing words when I say the work required to get the results you want will be tedious.

The final expectation I want to stress, although I've already stated this in a previous chapter, is the idea that your results are not long term. Again, you are losing water, not fat, and although no weight or fat loss program is long term if you don't stick to it, it is much easier for your body to start retaining water and for your weight to start creeping back up than it is for you to put back on actual fat – which requires a 3500 calorie surplus above your energy expenditure.

That's the brunt of it! If you thought there would be a lot more ominous warnings, I suppose you could call the above good news. If you are already freaking out about everything I have just stated and doubting whether you should proceed, don't fret. It's hard work for sure, but not impossible or not nearly as difficult as losing stubborn body fat.

Perhaps you can find some solace and encouragement in the fact that the results will be drastic, rapid and over before you know it (especially if you are doing the one day programs). That being said, we've reached the precipice of the background and groundwork, and can now move on to the actual programs and tasks ahead.

CHAPTER 6

NUTRITION OVERVIEW

As with typical fat loss, nutrition is the crux of how much water weight you can expect to lose and how good you will feel while losing it. The idea that you need to starve yourself to death to lose water weight is a myth.

Sure, an occasional fast, also known as intermittent fasting, of up to seventy-two hours won't do any damage – and we get into more details later on in the book on the best ways to fast - but when you start to get into four or more days of no food or calorie containing beverages, you are just setting yourself up for an increased likelihood to binge or make yourself feel faint and sick once everything is said and done.

That being said, it should go without saying that you cannot just eat whatever you like in unlimited qualities if you want to lose water weight, or any weight for that matter. The first reason is because every morsel of food has a weight that will contribute to your overall scale weights.

Other reasons include certain foods leading to more water retention and stoking the appetite more than others, and probably most obvious, if you eat at a calorie surplus (consume more calories than you expend) you will actually store fat and gain weight. Remember, all things considered calories in and calories out still come into play.

In the next few chapters we will go over the best and worst foods to get the water stuck in your system flowing and out of the body. Of course, if you'd like to preserve the results of this short term diet as long as possible it would behoove you to adopt and avoid the foods I am about to go over in your regular diet.

The foods to avoid will cover the most common foods that people are allergic to and thus cause an inflammatory reaction in the body, as well as hidden items to watch out for that goes beyond the eat low carb dogma, although that is included. The foods to include in your diet will cover the most common anti-inflammatory, anti-bloat, and cleansing products you can and should introduce to your diet beyond the scope of water or veggies and fruits, although I would remiss if I didn't include these proverbial biggies.

Regarding the age old question of the best time to eat, and how often and how much food you should be eating, research shows that meal timing and frequency doesn't matter so much when it comes to losing weight, and while physical activity is more important for maintaining weight, calorie restriction is best for losing weight.

In other words, as long as you are at a sizeable calorie deficit at the end of the day, you'll succeed. However, you should be mindful that meal timing and how often you eat should be adjusted to fit your schedule and routine in the best way that will allow you stay on track. That is, if you typically are not hungry when you wake up in the morning, don't feel obligated to eat breakfast, and if you absolutely hate going to bed hungry, don't feel like your last meal of the day needs to be at 5pm.

That being said, something will have to give, especially if your current habit and routine has you eating all the time. If you like to eat five or six times a day, you will have to make each meal much smaller to ensure you hit your calorie target. Of course, feeling really unsatisfied after each meal isn't an appealing strategy for most.

If you want to eat right when you wake up and not go to bed hungry, depending on how big you like your meals, it might mean you will have a long stretch between and after lunch where you go without eating, or you only get to eat twice for the day.

You have the liberty of playing around with your eating schedule and the number of meals you have per day until you find something that you can do every day without pulling your hair out. This doesn't mean being uncomfortable or even a little bit hungry means something is wrong, particularly if you are used to eating a lot of all the wrong foods all the time.

The body has an uncanny way of adapting relatively quickly to new eating schedules and after a few days you'll find yourself feeling hungry around the times you train your body to expect food.

For the most part though, a calorie deficit is where you want to spend most of your time and energy focusing on. Of course, there are some other ways to manipulate calories to spur faster visible results and we'll cover those techniques in more detail, but for now let's talk about how much of a deficit you should aim for.

As much as I'd like to give you a specific number, because everyone wants specific, the exact calorie amount you consume will vary again depending on your weight loss time frame, age, gender, height and level of activity (exercise and non-exercise).

One thing I want you to do though is discard the dogma about not reducing your calories to less than 1200 for women and 1500 for men out the window. No, your body will not go into starvation mode and refuse to use fat for energy if you force it to. Do you see the poor folks in third world countries walking around obese because their body has entered the dreaded starvation mode?

This theory just doesn't make any sense. Yes, your metabolism does slow down a little after long and prolonged period of extreme calorie restriction, but that's not what we are going to be doing here. Remember, this book is all about the short game to get you where you want to be, after which time you will need to make changes.

Furthermore, even with tracking, many people still end up underestimating or under calculating their calories by 20%, so if you pad your number to account for this very likely error or margin, you will probably be closer to reaching your mark It's the whole aim for the moon and land amongst the stars concept.

CHAPTER 7

OFF–LIMIT FOOD AND DRINKS

Grains and Carbs

As I've mentioned in my other books, *"Bye-Bye Thunder Thighs"* and *"The Thigh Gap Hack"*, people have slammed the Atkins Diet in the past under the basis that the huge initial weight loss most dieters experience when they go low carb is as a result of water weight loss. For some reason, they don't hesitate to point this fact out, as though it were a bad thing.

In reality, this massive shedding of pounds is a good sign and is the driving spark that motivates Atkins followers to stay the course long enough to start to see real fat loss. If you'll recall from earlier, when we reduce our calorie consumption, particularly of carbohydrates, our body stops feeding off the store of glycogen (a mixture of carbohydrate and mostly water) in our muscle tissue and liver and starts feeding off of the stored body fat.

There is another added benefit of following a low carbohydrate diet, and this element makes all the difference between successful and unsuccessful dieters. As you may already know it's really hard to fight insatiable hunger and much easier to lose weight when you don't feel compelled to eat all the time. When you lower your carbohydrate consumption you are likely to experience a decreased appetite.

To explain how fewer carbs leads to a lowered appetite we have to get a little scientific. You see, our hunger increases because high glycemic, processed carbohydrates cause our bodies to produce very high levels of insulin, known to trigger an increase in our hunger. Carbs are only responsible for 23% of insulin secretion, protein 10%, fat zero.

If that weren't bad enough, the same high glycemic carbohydrates also decrease a hormone called glucagon that helps to normally control our hunger. Glucagon normally communicates to the brain about how much body fat we have stored. When we have a lot of body fat glucagon levels are elevated hereby suppressing our desire to eat and create more body fat, but when we eat highly processed carbs, glucagon levels are abnormally suppressed and we lose the body's most potent appetite suppressant, so you get a double whammy.

On top of all of this, research by Dr. Zane Andrews, a neuroendocrinologist with Monash University's Department of Physiology, found that appetite-suppressing cells are attacked by free radicals, created naturally in the body after eating, causing our neurons, known as POMC, to degenerate over time. POMC's kick in when we are full, but when they are attacked by free radicals and degenerate this affects our judgment as to when hunger is satisfied.

Dr. Andrew's findings are extremely relevant to us because he found the degeneration of the POMC's to be more significant following meals rich in carbohydrates and sugars. In other words, the more carbs and sugars you eat the more your appetite control cells are damaged, potentially causing you to consume more.

No doubt you are aware of the anti-grain movement happening across America as a result of the recent onslaught of research and books highlighting the damaging effect grains can have to the body and mind, especially if you have a gluten intolerance or sensitivity.

If not, the basis of the argument against grain is that Americans consume enormous amounts of it, too much - both directly and indirectly. To be clear, any food made from wheat, rice, oats, cornmeal, barley or another cereal grain is a grain product.

We eat grain in the form of breakfast cereal, bread, pasta, tortillas, baked products, as a component in many processed foods, and, of course, by itself (oatmeal and grits for example). Not only do we eat a lot of grain, but we feed the animals that are raised for meat consumption a lot of grains too. When we then eat those animals we are indirectly putting grains into our bodies.

There are multiple reasons grains are being demonized which span beyond the scope of weight. First, although it seems like humans have always eaten grains, grain consumption only began a measly 10,000 years ago after the Agricultural Revolution. Before that time, humans existed for a couple hundred thousands years without any regular consumption of grains and numerous studies have shown that human brain function and physical ability actually peaked just prior to the agricultural revolution.

Even if we concede that our great grand parents ate grains and were the picture of health with a slender body to boot, or that the bible brandished grains as *the staff of life*, the no-grain advocates will be quick to point out what we eat today are a blatant departure from the grains of yesteryear.

In just a mere 50 years, grains – wheat, in particular – have become a mutant species crafted by the hands of human intervention in the name of increased crop yields, resistance to drought, disease, and heat, as well as an end to world hunger. The accelerated evolution of wheat through hybridization is how grains have gone from probably okay in moderation to being a different breed of food brandished by the *New England Journal of Medicine* as the cause of 55 diseases.

One counter argument that if you are not a celiac grains are perfectly fine for you isn't as cut and dry as the grain proponents would have you believe either. According to gluten expert Dr. Thomas O'Bryan, seven out of ten people are sensitive to gluten, the toxic protein found in most grains with one study showing that 29% of asymptomatic people (people who are not celiac) nonetheless tested positive for anti-gliadin IgA in their stool.

Anti-gliadin IgA is an antibody produced by the gut, and it remains there until it's dispatched to ward off gliadin, a primary component of gluten. The only reason anti-gliadin IgA ends up in your stool is because your body sensed an impending threat – gluten. If gluten poses no threat, the anti-gliadin IgA stays in your gut.

Along with the aforementioned pitfalls of grain, there is also the issue of lectins, which seemingly cause leptin resistance. Leptin is the master hormone that regulates body fat and is produced by the body's fat cells. Leptin resistance is when there is plenty of leptin floating around but the brain doesn't see that it is there, so people think they are starving and keep eating even though they have more than enough energy stored. Grass seeds that contain leptin blockers include wheat germ agglutinin (WGA) in wheat, barley, rye and rice.

Phytates provide another mark against the purported benefits of grains. Phytates make minerals bio-unavailable, rendering the healthy vitamins and minerals we are told we should get from whole grains null and void.

Knowing the reason behind staying away from certain foods makes it a lot easier to adhere to your diet because doing things which we have strong beliefs and convictions about is not in line with human behavior. Besides, there are so many no-grain and gluten free options that taste delicious readily available to consumers today that it makes the switch even easier.

Of course, there is a small chance that even given all of the above evidence you don't find yourself feeling a deep-seated hatred towards carbs and grains. It can be difficult to change your perception of something that you have a longstanding relationship with, especially when that thing has addictive properties, as grains do.

If that is the case, hopefully simply knowing that lots of carbs will make your body retain water will stir you enough to pass on the bread, pasta and rice during the period of your weight loss. Thereafter, even if you just say no to grains 50% of the time your health will be better off and your waistline will thank you.

Whenever you are tempted to give in try to remember carbohydrates stored in the muscle weigh 18g per kg of muscle and 1g of these is linked to 3.5g of water. It should be easy to see why it's important for anyone trying to cut weight to keep his or her carb intake low. By doing this, you also deplete muscle glycogen (a source of energy) and keep your body in flush mode.

Sugar, Fruit, and Starches

We've discussed the harmful and bloating effect of carbs from the consumption of grains, but while you may be willing to drop traditionally high carb foods, if you are still eating fruit and other starchy foods because they are not highly processed or refined, while you may not be damaging your health per say, there is a very high chance that you may be stalling your weight loss.

To further clarify, carbohydrates are classified according to their structure and as such there are three main types: sugars, starches, and fiber. Therefore, all starches and sugars are carbohydrates, but not all carbohydrates are starches or sugar alone.

Starches and sugars provide your body with its main source of energy. They're all comprised of carbon, oxygen and hydrogen, which are organized into single units. Sugars contain just one or two of these units and are "simple," while starches and fibers have many units of sugar, making them "complex".

While on the topic of simple and complex, you might also have heard of simple and complex carbs referred to as good (complex) and bad (simple) carbs. The reason for the labels is because of the glycemic load of these foods, how easy they are to digest and the nutritional value to the body.

For example, complex carbohydrates are considered good because of the longer series of sugars that make them up and take the body more time to break down. They generally have a lower glycemic load, which means that you will get lower amounts of sugars released at a more consistent rate — instead of peaks and valleys —to keep you going throughout the day.

Simple carbohydrates are considered bad because the body breaks them down too quickly to provide an adequate source of nutrients, vitamins or energy. Bad carbohydrates are foods that are composed of refined or processed flours and often include added sugars. Simple carbohydrates included sugars such as fruit sugar (fructose), corn or grape sugar (dextrose or glucose) and table sugar (sucrose).

Does this mean that since fruit is a simple or bad carb, you shouldn't be eating copious amounts of it if you want to lose weight? The short answer is, yes. Table sugar and the sugar

71

found in your fruit are made up of the same two components: fructose and glucose.

In fact, the ratios of fructose and glucose are pretty much the same in both fruit and table sugar. Most fruits are 40 to 55 percent fructose (there's some variation: 65 percent in apples and pears; 20 percent in cranberries), and table sugar (or sucrose) is 50/50. When you think about it, why would your body process sugar with almost the exact same composition differently?

To answer question, it won't. The molecular structure and composition of sugar molecules is the same no matter where they come from meaning your body can't distinguish between the sugars founds in fruit and chips, cakes, pies and cookies. When you take sugar down to its chemical make up - fruit sugar and any other sugar all look the same.

On that note, it's not just fruit sugar and table sugar that you need to be wary of. For example, there are many other types of sugar: besides fructose (fruit sugar), there is lactose, which is found in milk, ribose, found in the RNA within your cells, and sucrose (commonly in the form of cane sugar) is a disaccharide composed of glucose and fructose.

Every single one of these sugars, as well as starches, are converted to glucose, commercially known as dextrose, before being completely metabolized within our cells. In other words the body treats all of the sugar the same way – raising insulin and attracting water weight.

To be clear, it's quite obvious that while the sugar is treated the same from fruits, milk, cookies or cake, these foods don't have exactly the same overall effect on the body. For one thing, fruit actually contain antioxidants, water and vitamins, while typical desserts don't offer anything by way of nutrition.

Additionally, there is less sugar by volume in fruit and more fiber, which actually slows down your body's digestion of glucose, so you don't get the crazy insulin spike and subsequent crash compared to standard sweet treats that make the simple sugar list.

The fiber in fruits and vegetables changes the way that the body processes their sugars and slows down their digestion, making them a bit more like complex carbohydrates. Finally, fructose breaks down in your liver and doesn't provoke an insulin response while glucose starts to break down in the stomach and requires the release of insulin into the bloodstream to be metabolized completely.

So when proponents of high fruit diets or fruitarians claim fruit will affect your blood sugar/insulin levels differently than a piece of candy because of the rate at which the sugar is digested/metabolized, they are right.

However, they are talking about nutrients plus sugar versus other sugar, while we are talking about sugar versus sugar. When it's the latter, from a caloric and therefore a strictly weight loss point of view, you will retain water from sugar – which is a carb, regardless of the source.

Unlike sugar, starch is made from molecules that are linked together in long chains. Because of these long chains, starches are sometimes called complex carbohydrates. However, as you now know, starches are a type of carbohydrate – so naturally if we are limiting high carbohydrate foods we need to limit starchy foods as well to lose water weight.

Foods high in starch include bread, cereal, pasta, crackers, starchy vegetables (green peas, corn, lima beans, potatoes), and dried beans (pinto beans, kidney beans, black-eyed peas and split peas.). As you can see, many foods considered healthy (vegetables and beans) fall into the high starch category.

Thankfully though, there are non-starchy, high fiber healthy food options that will help slow the digestion and absorption of carbohydrates, be low in calories and keep water retention at bay.

These options include spinach, artichoke, asparagus, bamboo shoots, bean sprouts, beets, brussels sprouts, broccoli, cabbage (green, bok choy, Chinese) carrots, cauliflower, celery, chayote, coleslaw (packaged, no dressing), cucumber, daikon, eggplant, greens (collard, kale, mustard, turnip), hearts of palm, jicama, kohlrabi, leeks, mushrooms, okra, onions, pea pods, peppers, radishes, rutabaga, salad greens (arugula, chicory, endive, escarole, lettuce, spinach, radicchio, romaine, watercress), sprouts, squash (crookneck, cushaw, spaghetti, zucchini), sugar snap peas, swiss chard, tomato, turnips, water chestnuts and yard-long beans.

Sweeteners

Most of us love having something sweet every now and then because sweet things not only tastes very good but also help us to relax, thanks to the taste of sugar which releases endorphins that calm us. This is the reason why sugar cravings are so common.

So when you're told you have to cut down on sugar to drop inches and pounds, it might be very temping to turn to artificial sugars and sweeteners thinking that this is better than the alternative to the credit of the marketing team for the artificial sugar industry.

You would be wrong, but hardly alone or at fault, as the belief that artificially sweetened foods and beverages will help you lose weight is a carefully orchestrated deception. Many people, including diabetics – who are put even more at risk because aspartame has been shown to worsen insulin sensitivity, have been duped into thinking this way.

The truth is that research has repeatedly shown that artificial no or low calorie sweeteners are anything but good news for weight loss. Contrary to popular belief, studies have found that artificial sweeteners such as aspartame can: stimulate your appetite, increase carbohydrate cravings, and stimulate fat storage and weight gain.

In fact, a recent study[1] published in the January 2013 issue of the journal Appetite suggested that saccharin and aspartame caused greater weight gain when compared to sucrose (sugar) despite total caloric intake amongst all groups in the study being similar. The explanation was that a decrease in energy expenditure or increases in fluid retention were the culprits.

Notable points worth mentioning in the study involves the way your body reacts to artificial sweeteners – that is sweet taste, regardless of caloric content, enhances your appetite. Apparently when your body gets the sweet taste provided by artificial sugars, without the calories to go with it, it adversely affects your appetite control mechanisms, causing your food cravings to be increased.

---

[1] Appetite January 1, 2012, Volume 60, Pages 203-207

Conversely, the calories in natural sweeteners trigger biological responses to keep your overall energy consumption constant, leading to lower food consumption when compared to non-caloric artificial sweeteners. In this instance, natural sugar has the upper hand but honestly, it's just the lesser of two evils for losing weight fast.

Additionally, as alluded to briefly before, another reason for the potential of artificial sugars to cause weight gain is because the two acids that make up artificial sugars like aspartame (phenylalanine and aspartic acid) are known to rapidly stimulate the release of insulin and leptin.

In other words, although you're not getting the calories in the form of sugar, your body is reacting as though you have consumed sugar by raising your insulin and leptin levels, which in turn prevents your body from burning fat and promotes fat storage. Prolonged use can cause leptin resistance, which will leave you feeling hungry all the time, craving sweets and storing even more body fat.

It should be pretty clear by now, but just to be sure the moral of the story is not only should you stay away from natural sugar during your crucial weight loss period, but you should definitely not turn to artificial sweeteners for respite. You'll have to use good old-fashioned restraint, discipline and a strategic plan (upping protein and fats) to break your addiction to sweets.

Salt / Sodium

While carbs/starches and sugars aren't automatically associated with water weight gain, the exact opposite is true for salt and sodium. The health food organizations have done a great job of drilling into our heads the dangers or ill effect of too much salt, one of them being water retention, but those same organizations do have a track record of getting things wrong in the past (e.g. promoting high carb and low fat dietary guidelines).

Now, obviously I've listed salt and sodium in the foods to avoid category so you might not think much will be revealed that you don't already know. Not so fast, because I've got news for you. Reducing sodium and salt is not a one hundred percent foolproof way to lose water weight. In fact, the exact opposite can occur if you don't trek wisely.

Now, before we begin our discussion about salt/sodium and how it relates to water weight it is necessary to define in no uncertain terms the difference between the two since they are often used interchangeably.

Table salt or sodium chloride is added to food during cooking and at the dinner table to enhance the flavor of our food, or to return flavor to processed foods and help preserve them.

Sodium is what we look at in the nutritional content of a food. It is found naturally in most foods and accounts for approximately 40% of table salt. Therefore, when salt is added to food, the sodium content increases by approximately 40% of the amount of salt added.

The body can't function without sodium. Period. The function of sodium in the body is to bind water and maintain intracellular and extracellular fluids in the right balance. It is also an electrically charged molecule that along with potassium, helps maintain electrical gradients across cell membranes, which is critical for nerve transmission, muscular contract and various other functions

If sodium, the stuff found naturally in most foods, is critical to our well being it stands to reason that salt (the stuff we add to our food) is what we need to examine in relation to our diet. You would be correct, so let's get in to just how much salt/sodium you need under what circumstances now.

Salt is quite interesting because it does not cause your body to gain or lose fact. In fact, salt has absolutely no calories. High consumption of salt only results in temporary weight gain as it causes your body to retain water. Conversely, low

79

consumption of salt can result in temporary weight loss as it causes your body to expel water.

When I say only, note that I am not undermining this effect, as retaining water is something that is definitely of valid concern to those of you reading this book. The above certainly doesn't mean that salt is of little importance. To the contrary, salt should be of very high concern in regards to long term weight loss because not only can a diet high in salt content affect your blood pressure and temporary water weight, it is typically associated with gain beyond water weight.

The reason is because salt or sodium is most prevalent in processed foods that are high in calories, low in fiber and yes, even high in sugar. Think about the meals you would find in fast food chains, restaurant meals and TV dinners on your supermarket shelves.

Since the diet of most Americans is mostly made up of these highly processed foods, the intake of salt is through the roof, along with the number of calories. Just how bad is it? According to the Mississippi State Department of Health, most Americans consume on average 3,436 mg (about 1.4 teaspoons) of sodium per day, more than twice the daily-recommended amount. More than 75% of that sodium is from processed and restaurant foods[2].

---

[2] Mattes RD, Donnelly D. Relative contributions of dietary sodium sources. J

That being said, contrary to conventional nutrition recommendations, the answer is not as simple as forgoing processed foods and completely removing sodium and salt in the diet altogether.

As I alluded to earlier, completely eliminating salt and sodium from the diet can actually increase water retention in the long term and cause you to pull your hair out in frustration when you expected different results. On the other hand, short-term (meaning up to three day) stints of sodium reduction are effective.

Here's why – blood volume, which is governed primarily by sodium, carbon dioxide and serum albumin along with certain minerals such as potassium, magnesium and calcium, and hormones, like progesterone, renin, aldosterone and oestrogen, needs to be properly maintained in order to keep cellular fluid retention in check.

If you don't have enough sodium from dietary salt and are guzzling water (as many people are wont to do), serum albumin is unable to keep water from leaving the blood and entering the tissues, causing tissue water retention, and vice versa.

Am Coll Nutr. 1991;10:383–93.

Remember, sodium is a crucial electrolyte in the body and in the diet it helps to increase active thyroid hormone and metabolic rate, increase the production of protective carbon dioxide (CO_2), and restrain stress hormones and inflammation.

Meanwhile, carbon dioxide regulates the movement of calcium and sodium into and out of the cell by buffering cellular pH in the form of carbonic acid. In a low metabolic state (i.e. - hypothyroidism) carbon dioxide production is deficient and salt is excessively excreted, both contributing to the retention of water and puffiness.

So, to answer the big question of exactly how much sodium/salt you should have to keep water weight at bay, as with everything, it varies according to where you are starting as an individual and whether you are aiming for long term versus short term results.

In the long term overall balance is key. You want to keep your sodium intake moderate without completing ridding it from your diet. In the short term, reducing sodium intake to very low amounts (for example, 1,000 to 1,500 milligrams daily) would likely result in a loss of about 600 milliliters (2.5 cups) of water on the first day or about 1.25 pounds (.57 kilogram) of scale weight. Over a seven-day period the total loss of water weight from substantial sodium reduction is likely to be about 3 pounds (1.4 kilograms).

For a longer-term strategy, while the major health organizations don't all quite agree on an exact number, their recommendations suggest we should aim for less than 1500mg of sodium per day and definitely not more than 2300 mg:

- United States Department of Agriculture (USDA): 2300 mg.
- American Heart Association (AHA): 1500 mg.
- Academy of Nutrition and Dietetics (AND): 1500 to 2300 mg.
- American Diabetes Association (ADA): 1500 to 2300 mg.

To be clear, just because you don't need to completely give up all salt does not give you a pass to go from a low to high salt intake, especially if you need to lose water weight fast.

I cannot stress enough that when sodium is consumed in food nearly one hundred percent of the sodium is absorbed, so water will be temporarily retained until the body can reestablish sodium and water balance by excreting excess sodium and water in the urine at the expense of continued retention of sodium and water.

To those of you who are starting with high levels of salt and worry about your food tasting bland, simply replace excess salt with herbs and spices such as garlic, ginger, turmeric, black pepper, chives, cilantro, cayenne pepper, basil, oregano, or anything else your taste buds desire.

Read labels of your foods and snacks to confirm you don't go above your daily-recommended limits. Finally, be sure to also get adequate complete protein as serum albumin is a marker of dietary protein and good metabolism relies on getting enough, without overdoing it, dietary protein).

Alcohol

Over the last few years there have been a good amount of research and press dedicated to the benefits of red wine and other alcohol. I hate to be the bearer of bad news, but you'll have to choose between wine or your waistline because the purported positive effects of alcohol does not translate over to dieting and losing weight fast.

Drinking alcohol, whether in the form of wine, liquor, or beer, can impede weight loss for numerous reasons, from what it does to your metabolism to how it alters your mood to the calorie contents of the alcohol and other ingredients accompanying your drink. Don't just take my word for it though, the correlation between weight gain and alcohol has been proven by the countless studies showing people who drink alcohol on a diet have a harder time losing weight than those who do not drink at all.

The first thing that should give you reason for pause before dismissing the idea that you could ever give up alcohol, is that alcohol is known to negatively affect your metabolism. The reason has to do with the way it is handled in the body.

The metabolic process is your body's act of turning food and drink into other compounds that, ultimately, our body uses for energy. Throwing a wrench into your metabolism like alcohol means your body can't absorb the proper energy source it needs for day-to-day functions.

Since your body can't store calories from alcohol for later, the way it does with food calories, when you drink your metabolic system must stop what it's doing (like, burning off calories from your last meal) to get rid of the booze. The result is that whatever you recently ate gets stored as fat.

Studies show that even small amounts of alcohol have a large impact on fat metabolism. For example, The New England Journal of Medicine published the results of a Swiss study showing that if you're on a 1250 calorie diet and get just 250 of those calories from alcohol, it can slow your metabolism by 36%.

Given how important an elevated metabolism is in relation to losing weight (an elevated and faster metabolism means you can eat more and/or lose weight faster) I would say this is one of the best reasons, if any, to place alcohol on your list of things to avoid.

Also hindered by alcohol is the body's ability to burn fat. Since alcohol and fat are both processed in the liver, when the liver is processing alcohol it cannot effectively metabolize fat. This forces the body to prioritize one over the other, and as alcohol is seen as a toxin that the body wants to be rid of right away, it takes precedence.

Third, we all know alcohol is a depressant, meaning even if you may feel better directly after drinking it; the ultimate end result is a somber, lethargic, and depressing mood. To that point, feelings of fatigue increase with alcohol consumption making you less likely to exercise and deceases your resolve to stick to your weight loss program.

Now since alcohol itself is metabolized mostly in the liver and kidney, not in the intestines where normal digestion occurs (meaning that it is almost never fully metabolized) there is some debate about whether alcohol calories count. For what it's worth, alcohol has 7 calories per gram, making it the second-most calorie-dense macronutrient. (That's just below pure fat, which has 9 calories per gram. Carbs and protein have 4 calories per gram.)

However, even if you don't subscribe to the belief that alcohol calories count, the other stuff added to the alcohol that makes your drink taste good does get metabolized (namely, sugar and carbohydrates) and can lead to weight gain in the form of a calorie surplus. Given your newfound in depth knowledge about the detriments of sugar, carbs and alcohol, this triple whammy is a big no-no.

If you per chance are thinking that you'll just sacrifice a meal for a drink, consider that research has shown a 20% increase in calories get consumed at a meal when alcohol was consumed before the meal. Blame it on the lowered inhibitions or impaired judgment, but in studies, people who drank alcohol with their meals consumed a total of 33% more calories, so your intention to swap out food for alcohol probably won't go over as well as planned.

Finally, alcohol acts as a diuretic, which can lead to dehydration that makes the body hold on to fluids. Also related to dehydration, the morning after a night of imbibing has been known to leave many with cravings for large amounts of cheesy, greasy, fast food. Part of the problem is that when people feel dehydrated, as they do after drinking, they often mistake their need for water with hunger and give in to the nearest diner or fast food joint that promises satisfaction.

If you are not much of a drinker, count your lucky stars, as the biggest culprit for consuming alcohol is social situations and peer pressure from friends and/or family. Just because you are no longer consuming alcohol though doesn't mean you can't go out and have a social life. I've found that explaining that you're abstaining from alcohol because you are watching your weight can lead to pointless debates where people will bring up the talking points they overheard on the news regarding one glass being good for you, or alcohol calories not counting.

However, you now know the ugly truth and can see the forest for the trees – the big picture on how alcohol truly inhibits your goals. Feel free to borrow from my own arsenal of canned responses for when I am offered alcohol and questioned when I decline.

Simply state that you have to get up early the next morning to do something important, remind your companions that you've driven and you don't want to risk it, blame a medication you're taking (a lot of prescriptions require laying off alcohol in order to work effectively), or cite a headache and stomachache as a result of drinking or as a reason why you shouldn't. This should get everyone off the subject or off your back and leave you free to enjoy the night out while staying on your weight loss track.

CHAPTER 8

ANTI-BLOAT FOOD AND DRINKS

I admit the amount of food and drink items that are off limits when you are dedicated to moving the scale in short order is a long one, but I implore you to not get discouraged. As you will soon see, the list of anti-bloat foods and drinks designed to help trim you down is equally as long and appealing to your natural taste buds once you cleanse your hypersensitive palette.

Might I add, that the foods that we are about to cover will not only aid you in shedding weight, but promote glowing, tighter skin, lead to mounds of energy, and aid towards a body composition most people find desirable – to name a few of the added benefits.

High Antioxidant Foods

Antioxidants are chemical compounds found in plants, including beans, nuts, seeds, grains – and even meat, dairy products and eggs (which mainly stem from the nutrient rich plants the animals fed on), and in our bodies that inhibit oxidation or "rusting" of the cell. Oxidation is the beginning of the deterioration process – think about how a slice of apple turns brown when exposed to air.

Oxidation leads to the formation of free radicals, which are unstable molecules in the body that have one unpaired electron. To clarify, free radicals aren't necessarily villains – for example, immune cells will shoot free radicals onto invading bacteria in order to kill them.

In other words, free radicals are an important part of the body's defenses. However, too many free radicals – which can be taken into your body by inhaling smoke and other environmental pollutants, applying products to your skin that contain toxic chemicals, eating foods that contain chemicals, taking steroids and by exposure to radiation – where your normal antioxidant defenses become overwhelmed, leaving you vulnerable to cell damage and disease is when they become problematic.

Most people realize that antioxidants play a large role in preventing and fighting disease, but what is not so widely known is the role they play in maintaining your goal weight and even losing fat/weight.

According to a study in the *Journal of Agricultural and Food Chemistry,* antioxidants reacted with fat cells in mice to cut the cells' production of triglycerides— which are needed for energy, but can raise the risk of heart disease when

91

overproduced, as is common in people with extra body fat. Of course more research is needed, but these findings have uncovered an exciting development in weight loss, while simultaneously confirming the positive effects of a diet rich in antioxidants.

Another no-brainer reason to seek out foods rich in antioxidants is because they are some of the lowest calorie and contain qualities (nutrient dense) that make them ideal for promoting weight loss. One of the keys behind weight loss is consuming foods that help fill you up while providing few calories, and are rich in fiber.

Most fruits, vegetables and other fiber-rich plant foods, which also happen to be full of antioxidants, are ideal for controlling your calorie intake, promoting good health and defending against disease. Besides this fact, a very real correlation exists between eating the best, most nutrient dense foods and feeling strong, focused and empowered to continue to eat healthfully.

Further, some of these antioxidant rich foods directly correlate to weight loss. For example, the cathechins in green tea are known to stimulate the body to burn calories and decrease body fat, the pectin found in lemon peels has been shown to aid weight loss (lemon water), and grapefruit helps your immune system and is considered to be an ideal fat burner.

Additionally, once the body has consumed the foods that contain these high levels of antioxidants, the body is able to reduce the toxins within the body. Sometimes, it is the toxins within the body that are responsible for the water weight gain or fluid retention that can occur in the body.

Toxins are stored in fat cells. If your body is not making enough antioxidants and you aren't eating enough foods high in antioxidants then your body may hold on to the fat you are storing simply as a defense mechanism. It is preventing you from being flooded with these toxins. This will slow your metabolism and you may notice that you are stuck on a plateau with your weight loss even when you aren't eating much.

Toxins can even affect your brain chemistry (neurotransmitters) interfering with appetite control and proper hormone regulation. So how do antioxidants work to help you with this? When you are eliminating your body's waste with the help of enough antioxidants they are improving your biochemistry and helping your metabolism to work efficiently. Getting enough antioxidants will also help you to control your blood sugar levels.

That being said, before you run out to the nearest vitamin store to stock up, you should know that if your intention is to lose weight, your antioxidants should come from whole foods. This advice comes from the results of a 2009 German study, which found that when exercisers took antioxidants supplements (vitamins C and E), they weren't rewarded with the typical post exercise boost in insulin sensitivity. Therefore, to get your fill of antioxidants, look to the following foods instead of pills:

Vitamin A, and precursors known as carotenoids, can be found in carrots, squash, broccoli, sweet potatoes, kale, tomatoes, and apples.

Vitamin C can be found in citrus fruits like oranges and lemons, bell peppers (any color), leafy greens, strawberries and tomatoes.

Vitamin E can be found in leafy greens, avocados, broccoli, squash, and even in nuts and seeds like sunflower seeds.

Selenium is mostly found in meat products such as red meat and chicken, eggs, fish and shellfish.

Lycopene can be found in tomatoes, pink grapefruit and watermelon.

Protein and Fat

If you have to avoid carbs, sugar, salt and starches, you may be wondering if you'll have to eat air pie to meet your weight loss goals. I've got great news for you. No, you don't have to starve. You are allowed to eat what's left after you remove the above, and that leaves us with protein and fat.

Lean meats (chicken, fish, turkey), eggs, or a vegetarian source of protein (soy, tofu), leafy vegetables (spinach, arugula, kale, cabbage, etc.), and cruciferous vegetables (broccoli and cauliflower) will be the primary items on your menu during your cutting period.

I cannot stress enough that you cannot have unlimited quantities of these foods even though they are good for you and not calorie dense. Despite claims and recommendations by other weight loss plans, anyone is entirely capable of eating so much vegetables and so-called healthy, good or nutritious foods that they exceed their calorie requirements.

Just think of all the overweight vegans, vegetarians and fruitarians struggling to lose weight out there. Even if you personally don't know any, I'd encourage you to do a quick internet search and you'll see the phenomena truly exists and is actually very common due to people buying into the poor advice that they can consume unlimited healthy foods.

Remember, you don't want to undo all your work to drop weight by eating at a calorie surplus, which is bound to result in you gaining weight so track and weigh every morsel of food. There is no set amount of grams of protein or fat that you need to consume, but since fat has 9 calories per gram versus protein's 4 calories per gram, you might want to aim for 50% protein and 30% fats.

Studies actually show that diets too high in fat (especially saturated fats) actually blunt satiety signals and due to the excess calories, can cause unwanted fat gain

Caffeine

There's a pervasive and recognizable notion of slender NYC runway models subsisting on coffee and cigarettes to help maintain their figures. The reason for the common combination is the nicotine in cigarettes acts as both a stimulant and a depressant - which is one reason why it is so addictive. It calms the nerves while creating a rush of energy, and has a mind-clearing effect similar to caffeine, therefore the more you smoke, the more you want – even more than food.

With a suppressed appetite as well as hands and mouths that are constantly occupied that would otherwise be scarfing down food you get weight loss. As for the coffee, it sends the drinker running to the restroom often enough to keep any hint of water weight at bay.

While I would never suggest taking up smoking or discourage you from quitting just to realize the appetite suppressing qualities of nicotine as it is incredibly hard to kick because it is both physically and psychologically addictive, for the coffee fans and lovers among you, you may be happy to hear you may not have to give up your prized drink for eternity in exchange for your dream body.

When people talk of coffee helping to keep weight off, specifically they are referring to the caffeine that makes coffee a diuretic. A diuretic is any substance that promotes the production of urine (this includes forced diuresis) and helps rid your body of salt and water.

They work by making your kidneys put more sodium into your urine. The sodium, in turn, takes water with it from your blood. That decreases the amount of fluid flowing through your blood vessels, which reduces pressure on the walls of your arteries.

How much the diuretic effects from caffeine will apply to you will depend on variables such as personal tolerance, weight, and age. Other variables include just how much caffeine your particular type of coffee contains and how much coffee you actually drink.

If you are a caffeine naïve individual – meaning you don't normally drink coffee, and you have a couple of strong cups of caffeinated coffee in the morning, then you are probably going to need to use the restroom a little more often, and with greater urgency, than you normally do.

It should go without saying then that the more coffee/caffeine you drink and the higher your tolerance, the less the effect you will see. This is because the body develops a tolerance to caffeine after about three to five days of regular use – which greatly diminishes the weak diuretic effect of caffeine. In other words, you don't want to overdo it by chugging coffee down morning, noon, and night if you want to get the most kick out of using caffeine for water weight loss purposes.

It's also worth addressing the other side of the coin – the idea that caffeine should not be used as a diuretic due to the risk of dehydration. This once believed myth has been put to rest with the most recent studies declaring caffeine to not typically cause dehydration. In fact, according to the Mayo Clinic, "While caffeinated drinks may have a mild diuretic effect they don't appear to increase the risk of dehydration".

However, I must warn those of you who have heard about pure caffeine powder and are contemplating using it to supplement your weight loss – perhaps because you don't like the taste of coffee or whatever reason you may have, you may want to reconsider.

Just one teaspoon of pure caffeine powder is the equivalent to twenty-five cups of coffee, meaning just a small amount can cause an accidental overdose. Therefore, stick to the small quantities found in coffee, as some teas, or forget using caffeine for diuretic purposes altogether.

Water

Right off the bat, let's dispel the notion that water has some magical property that burns fat. Sorry, it doesn't work that way. The good news is water consumption is directly correlated with weight loss – even beyond short-term water weight loss. The bad news is if you don't know what you're doing it's possible to overdo water consumption and/or end up bloated and heavier than your liking because your body won't let go of the water you consume.

The first of many ways drinking water positively affects your ability to lose weight is by preventing overeating. Since hunger is a symptom of dehydration many people are guilty of mistaking their feeling of thirst for hunger and compensate by eating. Thus a glass of hydrating h20 could save you many unnecessary calories if you turn first to the drink instead of food whenever your tummy rumbles.

The water should either quench your actual thirst and quell hunger pangs or at least allow you to stave off raving the fridge for thirty minutes, at which time if you still feel hungry you would know it's not just phantom hunger. Additionally, you could keep drinking water and use it as a distraction to keep you from eating between meals.

Water can also help you consume fewer calories in your diet overall, thus enabling you to lose weight, by literally filling your stomach up so there's less space for food. This is called pre-loading and was studied by associate professor of nutrition at Virginia Tech, Brenda Davy, Ph.D.

The study included 48 overweight or obese men and women between the ages of 55 and 75 who were on a low-calorie diet (1,200 calories per day for women and 1,500 calories per day for men). Half of the people were instructed to drink 16 ounces of water -- the amount in a small bottle of spring water -- before meals.

After three months, the participants who drank water had lost an average of about 15.5 pounds, compared with just 11 pounds in the control group, according to the study, the first results of which were published earlier this year in the journal Obesity.

It makes perfect sense when you think about it. When you are so full that taking another bite of food causes you to feel discomfort, you will find it much easier to put the fork down and push the plate away.

To pre-load, simply drink a large glass or two of water at least twenty minutes before every meal (not during because water dilutes digestive juices and minimizes absorption of the nutrients) as a way of forced portion control adherence that doesn't solely rely on your will power.

An added tip is to bring a refillable water bottle with you everywhere you go, to work, to the park, to the gym, to meet friends, etc. and drink from it throughout the day. This way you'll always be armed should you start to feel hungry or find yourself in an unplanned situation to eat. Plus, sipping steadily in small amounts throughout the day trumps chugging a large amount of water in one go, as the latter doesn't provide your body with the water it needs because that "flood" of fluid gets passed on to your bladder and only a slight amount is absorbed by your body.

Next, drinking water more than likely means you're not drinking something else – such as sugary, caloric beverages or potentially diet-breaking soda. Again, this is a way of ingesting fewer calories, which according to the law of thermodynamics, leads to weight loss.

Of course it might seem too obvious to point out, but it's worth mentioning that water hydrates your body. What does that have to do with losing weight, you ask? With proper hydration you get optimal organ function, keep your metabolism at optimum levels and more energy to do more activities, which in turn leads to more calories burned and puts your body in a better position to lose weight. Conversely, being dehydrated will slightly lower your metabolic rate.

I would be remiss if I didn't include an effective hack used by dieters that involve cold water to assist in weight loss. Lest you think it's too good to be true, science has given the theory validity with studies. Fir example, German researchers found that drinking 6 cups of cold water a day (that's 48 ounces) can raise resting metabolism by about 50 calories daily—enough to shed 5 pounds in a year. The increase may come from the work it takes to heat the water to body temperature.

Though the extra calories you burn drinking a single glass don't amount to much, making it a habit can add up to pounds lost with essentially zero additional effort as your body automatically does the work in converting ice-cold water to body temperature by speeding up your metabolism.

This goes beyond superficial water weight since your metabolism is actually being sped up and you are burning calories. It makes sense then to kill multiple birds with one stone (hydrate your body, keep hunger at bay, feel full between meals, get more energy, consume fewer calories) and rev up your metabolism by drinking a few glasses of cold water daily.

Finally, and most importantly for those who want immediate results, drinking water helps your body get into flushing mode. It can seem confusing and downright counterintuitive to drink more water to get your body to release water, but the fact of the matter is our bodies sometimes works in mysterious and counterintuitive ways.

When you don't get enough water, your body panics and holds on to it selfishly as though you were in a famine as a defense mechanism against dehydration. That is because while our bodies can store energy as glycogen, fat, and tissue, it cannot store water. The body uses its own water but expects us to contribute by providing a continuous supply of fresh new water regularly. That being said, it might be more helpful to explain the step-by-step process so that you get a full picture of how consuming more water actually helps the body to flush retained water and help us lose weight.

To begin, water helps your liver convert fat into usable energy. If you don't drink enough, your kidneys are overwhelmed with concentrated fluids, and they will make your liver do extra work. Your liver works hard to turn your body fat into the energy that you use but if it has to do the kidney's work, then it simply holds onto the extra fat that would have been burned off if you only had enough water.

Water is also critical in moving nutrients into and out of a cell, an action known as the "ion pump". When you take in the improper balance of sodium and potassium or do not drink adequate water, your body will increase a hormone and try to "retain" water by keeping your kidneys from filtering it. Ironically, one of the best ways to stop retaining water is to drink more water.

However, drinking knocking back a few bottles of water in one go isn't the solution to get your body into this state, contrary to popular belief. When too much water floods your system all at once, your body will pass most of it on to your bladder, and only absorb a slight amount. Weight in the stomach is a signal for digestive processes to begin, and a number of biological chemicals enter your stomach and change the pH balance. This can result in indigestion and stomach pain.

While increasing your overall water intake will help your body let go of the water retention, there is an advanced and methodical strategy you can use to consuming water over the course of a week leading up to your big event that goes beyond the advice of simply drinking more water.

It involves starting at high levels of consumption, (one to two gallons of water a day depending on your activity level) and steadily decreasing the amount of water to hardly any at all up to the day you need to weigh in, fit into that dress or attend that event. As previously mentioned, you don't want to chug the water as much as you want to steadily sip it throughout the day.

By drinking lots of water early on, the body will down-regulate aldosterone, a hormone that acts to conserve sodium and secrete potassium. And when you suddenly reduce the amount of water you drink your body will still be in flushing mode, meaning you'll be running to the bathroom to pee a lot even though you're hardly consuming any water.

Now that you know you need to increase the amount of water you drink, the next logical question is what type of water you should choose? With all the brand options, and marketing message - tap water, bottled water, filtered water, distilled water, etc., it can be confusing and downright overwhelming to determine which water is truly the best and safest choice. It doesn't have to be that way though. The following section serves to demystify what kind of water you should and should not drink moving forward. First, let's have a look at the most common types of water readily available to us.

Tap water is municipal water that comes out of the faucets and has been treated, processed and disinfected. It is purified with chlorine and generally has added fluoride. It is considered generally safe if it comes from a public water system in the United States, such as one run and maintained by a municipality. The Environmental Protection Agency (EPA) has the authority to monitor all public water systems and sets enforceable health standards regarding the contaminants in drinking water.

Distilled water can be any kind of water that has been vaporized and collected, leaving behind any solid residues, including minerals. Distilled water has no minerals in it at all. Because it is devoid of minerals, distilled water grabs and holds onto minerals in the body, a process called chelation.

Distilled water can be used for a few months to remove toxic metals and toxic chemicals from the body quite effectively. Drinking distilled water for longer than this, however, always results in vital mineral deficiencies. Examples of distilled water include SmartWater and Sparkletts.

Deionized water has had ionized impurities and minerals removed from it but not bacteria or pathogens.

Reverse osmosis water has been forced through membranes that remove larger particles, pollutants and minerals. Reverse osmosis water is usually acidic and does not hydrate as well as spring water. Examples include Dasani.

All of the above water lack essential minerals that are necessary for good health. Mineral deficiency can lead to insulin resistance, migraines, high blood pressure, constipation and even heart beat irregularities so opting for water striped of its minerals is not the best choice you can make. Does that mean bottled water is your saving grace? Well, not quite.

Although marketed as being the purest option, and thus the most expensive of our available sources of drinking water, every bottle of water is not automatically so. Bottled water is often just purified municipal water that lack essential minerals. (Brands like Dasani and Aquafina are cleaned-up city water.)

Other brands like Sahara and Kirkland are actually just bottled tap water without anything done to it and is typically labeled as drinking water. Why anyone would pay for water he/she can get directly out of the tap, just bottled, boils down to simply not knowing that's what they are doing.

One of the major cons against bottled water is that dangerous toxins from some plastic water bottles can leach into your water. This can be avoided if you opt for bottled water in glass containers or transfer water to reusable glass containers.

To answer the original question, the best water you can drink is naturally clean and pure, full of naturally occurring minerals and is low alkaline, with a pH of 7.2 to 8, similar to our blood – although the tolerable pH as approved by the World Health Organization is 8.5 maximum.

Sources of water that fall within those categories include well water, spring water from a natural spring that is bottled at the source, artesian or spring waters from a natural source that is bottled off site after being processed and purified, or mineral water.

Spring water has been filtered by the earth in ways that works better than any invented means of purifying water and contains a wide variety of trace minerals the human body needs.

Artesian water is spring water that comes from a well that is dug in the earth that taps a confined aquifer - a water-bearing underground layer of rock or sand in which the water level is above the top of the aquifer. When dug, the internal pressure from the hole causes the water to burst forth spontaneously like a fountain. Examples include the brand, Fiji water.

Mineral water comes from an underground source and can include either natural spring water or artesian water. It contains no less than 250 parts per million total dissolved mineral solids and is defined by its constant level of mineral and trace elements at the point of emergence from the source. No minerals can be added to the water. Examples include Panna from Italy.

All of the aforementioned types of water have those necessary essential minerals and nutrients like magnesium, potassium and sodium that your body needs thereby making them the best water to drink. As for specific brands, Evian,

Volvic, Poland and Arrowhead Mountain Spring Water are good choices. Sure, they will be pricier than the generic brand at your supermarket, but as with most anything – you get what you pay for.

If obtaining these types of water proves difficult due to your location, home filters is the next option to look into. The main drawback regarding filters that you should be aware of is that while many filters, like Brita, remove chlorine and help clean your water, they also remove minerals.

As a result, be on the look out for filtration that utilizes ozonation, which does not change the mineral content of your water, and filtration that removes any particles that are larger than 1 micron in size. Again, the purpose is to leave minerals in the water.

While on the subject of filtration systems, there are some pretty pricey models out there that sing the praises of alkaline water (water that has been ionized to increase its pH to between 8 and 10) for its supposed antioxidant properties. Given what we know about the pH levels our drinking water should be, let's say that's strike one against alkaline water straight off the bat.

The second problem we need to address is that the purported antioxidant value of alkaline water only lasts for 18-24 hours after it's made, so bottling alkaline water makes no sense since the health benefits are gone in such a short period of time.

Strike three pertains to the way water is processed through the filtration system. Many of these devices pass tap water through a carbon filter leaving behind toxic metals and chemicals as the water must move quickly through the filter.

To make matters worse, the water then passes over electrified platinum and titanium plates to alkalinize it. The danger being that platinum and titanium are deadly toxic metals that can lead to platinum or titanium metal toxicity in users of these machines.

The verdict on these systems is to keep your hundred dollar bills safely tucked away in your wallet. You can alkalize the body in cheaper more effective ways such as drinking spring water, eating fresh foods and vegetables, and cutting out junk / processed foods from your diet. Alkaline water systems include the Jupiter, Kangen, I-Water and others.

In a perfect world you would be able to get the best water available, but you have to be realistic about the limitations of your environment and choose the best from what is accessible and affordable to you. For example, any filtration system is better than none at all and making sure you get adequate amounts of water is better than being nearly dehydrated due to decision paralysis on which brand to buy.

Foods with High Water Content

Naturally, if drinking lots of water can get your body to release water you might be curios about whether eating foods with high water content will similarly assist in flushing out your system. You would not be alone in drawing the parallels, and better still, you'd be right. The theory has been put to the test and confirmed by scientists.

In a University of Tokyo study, researchers concluded women who ate high-water-content foods had lower body mass indexes and smaller waistlines. When asked why, researchers speculated that the water in these foods fill you up so you eat less – one of the exact advantages to drinking more water named above.

Given the fact that many foods contain some water, I don't like vague instructions and the word high is pretty subjective, the specific amount of water content in food that constitutes being high in water content and that you should aim to include in your diet would be 80% and higher.

On top of the vegetables list are cucumber and lettuce, consisting of ninety-six percent water. There are many types of lettuce to choose from and iceberg lettuce is probably the most well known type, but it's also lacking any nutrients. Therefore, I would recommend dark green or purple lettuce as they contain the most nutrients and is a great source of B vitamins, folic acid and manganese, which helps regulate blood sugar and is essential for proper immune system function.

Zucchini, radish and celery are comprised of 95 percent water. While most of you will be familiar with zucchini and celery and well versed in the ways of preparing and consuming these vegetables, I've found many people are unfamiliar with and thusly missing out on the brightly colored radish.

This is a shame as radishes are packed with potassium, folic acid, antioxidants, and sulfur compounds that aid in digestion. One helpful preparation tip - don't make the mistake of discarding the leafy green tops, as they contain six times the vitamin C and more calcium than the roots.

Next on the list, pulling a double duty due to its ability to aid in metabolism is the tomato, which is made up of ninety-four percent water. Green cabbage follows with ninety-three percent water, while its cousin red cabbage clocks in at ninety two percent. Cabbage is rich in antioxidants like vitamin C and a great immune booster. Other vegetables that contain ninety-two percent water include eggplant and peppers.

Cauliflower is also ninety two percent water, full of phytonutrients and an excellent source of vitamin C and folate. It is also very versatile. To mention just a few of my favorite ways to prepare cauliflower: put it in the food processor and then light steam for five minutes over low heat to get what is referred to as cauliflower rice.

You can also cut cauliflower up into fine florets and add just a touch of olive oil before baking at 350 degrees for forty minutes to one hour. Sautéing it with other vegetables and a lean cut of protein, or grounding and mixing with egg white and other vegetables to create a makeshift grain and gluten free, pizza crust are two other ways I regularly enjoy this delicious vegetable.

Spinach, one of my favorite vegetables, also contains ninety two percent water, and is rich in iron, folic acid and vitamin K. Either raw as a salad substitute, lightly sautéed, added to egg whites and baked to form a quiche, or blanched and lightly seasoned, spinach can be filling and tasty.

Typically linked to cauliflower but just a teensy bit lower on the scale of water weight volume is broccoli at ninety one percent. Do I even need to mention it is a great source of fiber and calcium?

Broccoli is one of those foods that many of us decide we dislike at a young age more than likely because of the way our parents prepared it. For example, over cooked broccoli tends to get a squishy, rubbery texture and many people fail to season broccoli leaving it tasteless and flavorless. With the right recipe though, broccoli can taste mind-blowingly delicious.

If you want a recipe guaranteed to make you having broccoli cravings I recommend roasting them until they caramelize. Specifically, wash and cut broccoli into relatively big florets, dry them thoroughly, and toss with one tablespoon of olive oil per 6 ounces, pepper, garlic cloves, lemon juice, and lemon zest. Then place your well-seasoned broccoli on a cookie sheet and roast in the oven for twenty to twenty five minutes at 425 degrees until crisp-tender.

When it comes to fruits, there are plenty that have high water content. The problem lies in fruit's high sugar content. Too much sugar raises insulin levels, which in turn lessens the body's ability to expel sodium, and you should know what the result of too much sodium in the body results in by now. (See the previous chapter about off limit foods for a refresher)

The good news is that the fruits lowest in sugar are some of the highest in nutritional value, including antioxidants and other phytonutrients

To categorize, the fruits lowest in sugar according to the USDA database include small amounts of lemon or lime, rhubarb, raspberries, blackberries and cranberries (notice a theme here?) Out of this list, raspberries and cranberries alike contain eighty seven percent water weight, making them eligible to include in your diet of high water content foods.

Fruits low to medium in sugar include strawberries, casaba melon, papaya, watermelon, peaches, nectarines, blueberries, cantaloupes, honeydew melons, apples, guavas, apricots and grapefruit.

Winnowing down the field of options for only those fruits with high water content brings watermelon and strawberries to the front of the pack with about ninety two percent water per volume. Grapefruit has about ninety-one percent water and is refreshing and satiating as well as full of vitamin C, folic acid and potassium, and pectin.

Following closely behind grapefruit comes cantaloupe at ninety percent, and peaches with eighty-eight. Cranberries and raspberries are eighty-seven percent, apricots contain eighty six percent water volume, nectarines and blueberries tie for eighty-five percent and apples wraps things up at eighty-four percent.

Fruits fairly and very high in sugar, and thus should be excluded from your diet at least until you reach your goal weight / physique, are plums, oranges, kiwifruit, pears, pineapples, tangerines, cherries, grapes, pomegranate, mango, figs, bananas, and dried fruit.

High Potassium Foods

I've called out potassium rich foods throughout the book, but what is the relation between this mineral and weight loss or fluid retention?

Well, potassium is among the ten most common minerals in the body. It is essential for membrane polarization in the neurons of the nervous system, proper function of cells, tissues, and organs in the body. It is also required to maintain the osmotic balance between the cells and the interstitial fluids which put planning means it has a great deal to do with us having a normal water balance in the body. In fact, potassium deficiency is one of the main causes of water retention in the body.

As potassium regulates fluid balance and helps the kidneys to eliminate waste as well as help excrete excess water through urine we need to make sure we get adequate amounts of it. More specifically the number to aim for is 3,500 milligrams of potassium a day.

Potassium is available as potassium salts (chloride and bicarbonate). It is also present in various mineral chelates (aspartate, citrate, etc.) and food-based sources. However, since taking higher doses of potassium salts is risky and comes with adverse side effects such as nausea, vomiting, diarrhea and stomach upset, it is better to stick to water retention supplements or food sources (food sources does not cause negative side effects).

Reaching the recommended daily amount of potassium can be obtained by eating at least five servings of fruits and vegetables.

According to MedlinePlus, all meats are good sources of potassium, as are many vegetables, including broccoli, peas, potatoes, tomatoes, lima beans, spinach, raisins, sweet potatoes, beets, mushrooms, and winter squash. Potassium-rich fruits include prunes, kiwi, bananas, citrus fruit, cantaloupe and apricots. Other excellent sources of potassium include milk, yogurt and nuts.

Of course, I have to insert the obligatory word of caution here, at the risk of being redundant. Vegetables are the preferable choice over fruits when trying to move water weight due to the often times high sugar content of fruits. Don't hesitate to check back on the previous chapter to see the approved list of fruits and vegetables to cross reference lists about which foods are high in potassium so that you don't take two steps forward and one step back.

Once you've gotten your potassium rich foods sorted out, you need to be mindful of the way you prepare them. Potassium is lost in cooking water, so steam, grill or roast your veggies rather than boiling them. Finally, it's worth considering some of the more popular salt substitutes - NoSalt and Nu-Salt. These are potassium chloride and supply 530 milligrams of potassium per 1/8 teaspoon.

Garlic

Last but not least, garlic needs a special mention as one of the most effective natural diuretic food. First, a little history lesson: Garlic has been used for centuries throughout Europe, Asia and Africa as a popular seasoning as well as medicinal purposes.

Testimonials of its many health benefits have appeared in both the Bible and Talmud and it has been recognized in Chinese medicine for its healing powers for over 3,000 years. In India, 5,000 year-old Sanskrit records were found also singing the praises of garlic. With good press like that, there's got to be something to this tiny strong smelling, pungent tasting bulb.

Garlic not only helps in getting rid of excess water and toxins from the body, but also contributes to the breakdown of fats making it doubly effective in combating water retention and associated obesity. A moderate intake of fresh garlic is very effective home cure for water retention.

How about a little evidence to back up such lofty and bold claims? Laboratory tests showed that rats given a high sugar diet put on less weight if they were also given a garlic compound.

Not only is the evidence favorable in terms of weight loss, garlic has also proved effective in preventing high blood pressure, treating diabetes, curing diarrhea, lowering the risk of heart attacks and killing cancer cells. I like to say if garlic were a student it would certainly be in the running for valedictorian.

Of course given all of the benefits that come with eating garlic, it would be a shame if you unwittingly robbed yourself of its goodness by stripping it of its most desirable qualities during preparation or cooking.

Raw garlic needs to interact with the oxygen in air to form allicin, the active ingredient responsible for the garlic benefits. So, to clarify common beliefs about acceptable ways to consume garlic, you should know that cooking stops the process in which the active compounds in garlic are generated, but plenty are formed if you chop the garlic and allow it to stand for about 10 or 15 minutes before cooking it.

The only time cooking keeps us from getting garlic's health benefits is when we roast whole garlic, since the active compounds have not had time to form. That is still a healthy choice, since the soft cloves that result from roasting make a wonderful spread, with no fat or significant sodium.

The usual recommended dose is 700 to 1000 mg per day. That might seem like a lot if you are not used to eating garlic, but there are many ways to incorporate it into your food without dealing with an overwhelmingly garlic taste or garlic breath for that matter.

Some creative ways to sneak garlic into your food every day include adding it into egg white omelets or sautéing it with greens like cabbage, kale, or spinach. You can also cut in thin slices or smash and roast with brussels sprouts, cauliflower, broccoli or sweet potato, chop and drop into soups, mix it in to home made salad dressing, guacamole, hot sauce or honey lemon tea (this is strangely delicious), and of course use it as seasoning for chicken breasts or fish (I recommend salmon filets and raw or cooked tuna).

Fiber Rich Foods

Everyone says it because it is the truth - adding fiber to your diet will help your body get rid of those excess ions, water, and waste you're carrying around leaving you a few pounds lighter.

Our government recommends twenty-five grams of fiber per day for women under fifty, and teenage girls, and thirty to thirty eight grams of fiber daily for teenage boys and men under fifty. In comparison the American Cancer Society recommends twenty to thirty five grams of fiber per day, based on research indicating that higher fiber intake may reduce the risk of various forms of cancer.

Americans who eat the typical refined food diet only get about fifteen grams. Could there be a correlation to the obesity problem and the very low amounts of fiber being consumed by Americans? I'll let you speculate on that one.

There are two forms of fiber, water-soluble and water-insoluble. The main difference is soluble fiber dissolves in water, while insoluble fiber does not.

As it relates to weight loss, soluble fiber is probably the most important because it regulates the pace of calorie digestion and release into your bloodstream, which has a profound effect on insulin, blood glucose, and leptin. It also slows down digestion and keeps you feeling fuller longer. Approved sources of soluble fiber that fit into your water weight loss plan include cucumbers, celery, flaxseeds, beans, blueberries, psyllium, and carrots.

That doesn't mean that insoluble fiber is chopped liver though. Both types help weight loss by acting as a sponge for toxic waste, which is vital to get out during the weight loss process. Insoluble fiber are also considered gut healthy fiber because they add bulk to the diet, preventing constipation.

121

Since it doesn't dissolve in water they pass through the gastrointestinal tract relatively intact, speeding up the passage of food and waste through your gut.

Some approved sources of insoluble fiber are cabbage, broccoli, celery, zucchini, dark leafy vegetables, green beans, onions, tomatoes, and root vegetable skins.

Protein Energy Bars

Yes, you read that right – it is not a typo or an editing error that should have placed this in the section on off-limits foods. Allow me to provide you with some context before you lose all faith in me for promoting food that many instantly deem as glorified candy bars high in refined sugars, bad fats and other nasties.

While energy bars cannot take the place of a nutritious, meal, I would be like an ostrich with its head stuck in the sand if I did not face the reality that many of you will be forced to eat on the go due to our ever fast paced lives. As a result, I want to give you the best advice for when you are tempted to grab a bag of chips or greasy slice of pizza to hold you over. No, I don't condone snacking, but if you are going to snack here's the best things you can get.

Energy bars are convenient, travel well, and many are a good source of high quality protein. They provide a real energy boost that one might need when cutting calories, using heat therapy, or any of the other techniques in this book. In short, for a quick, small meal or snack on the go, they are the better choice than a fast food meal and other highly processed packaged convenient foods.

Additionally, they have a high calorie-to-weight ratio making them one of the best sources of calories in a food that only weighs a few ounces. This is perfect for eating around the time you need to look your best if you recall that everything you put in your mouth contributes to your final weight.

To be clear, this is not a pass to stock up on sugar filled candy bars (most containing chocolate and dried fruits) that are masquerading as healthy meal replacements when I suggest energy or protein bars.

Ideally, aim for bars with 15 grams or more of protein, at least 3 grams of fiber (the higher the better), and less than 30% of calories from sugar since many bars come in different weights and sizes. Other markers of a good bar include being low in saturated fat and no palm oil or other hydrogenated fats, or at least contain very small amounts of these fats (less than 2-3 grams or so for about 200 Calories of food).

Of course you want to make sure the calories are in line with your overall intake / deficit, but a slightly higher calorie content might be more desirable in your bar if this means it is more nutritious, containing less sugar and fat. After all, you don't have to eat the entire package all at once.

Some of the better bars on the market today are NuGo, GNU, Cliff Mojo and Odwalla. Don't even think about Think Thin, and the other very popular brands with enormous ingredient lists like Lara Bars, PowerBars or even the natural but very high sugar Kind Bars. New brands enter the space all the time though, so check out your natural food supermarket and be sure to read and analyze the labels *per serving* – this will give you the best overall picture of whether the bar is a hit or miss.

If you are having a hard time finding bars that meet your requirements, one option is to make your own. Believe it or not, it is not that hard to do and some don't even need to be baked – just mixed up the ingredients and pop them in the refrigerator for half hour.

This way you can control exactly what goes in it – or better yet, what doesn't go in it – like artificial colors/flavors, additives, and preservatives. When you are running the show, it's even easier to make sure nothing inflammatory like gluten, wheat, corn, dairy (if you're allergic), soy (found in almost every single food lately), sugar alcohols, which can cause intestinal discomfort, or any other undesirable ingredient that will lead to water retention, bloating or an impaired metabolism gets added.

Generally all you need is a base like coconut flakes, blended black beans, Bob's Red Mill gluten free oats or steel cut Irish oats, and flaxseed meal are a good place to start; something to bind all the ingredients together like applesauce, gelatin, coconut or almond milk, plain Greek yogurt (fat and sugar), egg white, or almond butter. For flavors consider fresh ginger, puréed pumpkin, vanilla, herbs used in teas, and spices like cinnamon, maca, all spice or nutmeg.

Nuts tend to be very high calorie and inflammatory for a lot of people, so you might want to look into seeds like pumpkin seeds, hemp seeds, sunflower seeds or chia seeds instead. For the kicker needed to make the protein bars palatable or taste a bit more appealing, opt for dates soaked overnight before chopping them in a food processor with the rest of the ingredients, or blueberries and raspberries instead of sugar or honey.

Just in case you didn't notice, I failed to mention protein powder and that was done on purpose. Have you ever actually read the ingredients on the back of those huge jugs of powders? Well, I'll spare you the waste of time and just say that commercial protein supplements contain dangerous chemicals and are highly processed.

As evidenced above, it is entire possible to use real foods and natural ingredients to make a nutritious and filling bar. So, even though you aren't cooking and eating a full meal when you grab one on the go, your body will still benefit from the stuff it naturally needs and knows how to properly digest. For some of my favorite recipes, check out the resources page on my website www.thighgaphack.com/resources.

Of course, these bars should not be used as a substitute for all your meals, and I generally disapprove of eating them as a morning breakfast substitute because the first thing you put in your mouth should be real food. Reserve your bar for lunch or dinner, especially if your prior meals have been comprised of nutrient dense whole foods.

CHAPTER 9

TOOLS AND RESOURCES

Besides nutrition and exercise, there are numerous other ways to manipulate your water weight in a short period of time. Some tools, gadgets and resources you may be familiar with and are quite easy or simple to access or implement, while other techniques will seem bizarre or require more effort to complete or withstand. Some I recommend using if you have a very short time frame to cut weight but caution against otherwise.

I will go through each technique one by one, but you should know that you are not required to do everything mentioned here altogether and in any specific fashion or order. Although, the more techniques you combine, the faster you will see results. When we get to the one day, seven day and two week plans, I will specifically recommend which tools and resources from the below list that you should use and when.

Think of the following list as a reference for everything that is available to you. If you are not pressed to lose a given amount of weight in a span of time feel free to thumb through this chapter and simply pick and choose any of the following.

Saunas

A sauna is a small room or house heated to about 150 to 194 degrees Fahrenheit, designed as a place to experience dry or wet heat sessions. It is thought of as a place for cleaning, relaxing and refreshing the body, and can typically be found in Banyas, spas or bathhouses.

The primary way in which saunas assist with water weight loss is by causing your body to overheat and sweat, which causes your body to work harder, your heart to pump faster, your metabolism to increase, and salt and water to be shed from the body.

Not all saunas are created equally; there are different types of saunas such as traditional saunas, far-infrared saunas and steam baths. No one is better than the other, but there are differences.

Traditional saunas are for those who enjoy steam in the sauna, higher temperatures and a more social environment, while far-infrared saunas generally have lower temperatures but with body penetrating heat. Additionally the traditional sauna will be drier (10% or lower) in humidity and is the only bath in the world where the user controls both the temperature and humidity, by sprinkling water over the rocks. In far-infrared saunas you control the temperature but the humidity is whatever it is.

The sauna you choose should be at least 150 degrees and you should spend up to 30 minutes at a time, with 20 minute being the optimum length per session. If you feel woozy or need a break sooner, that's fine but even if you're not, take a break and cool down every half an hour.

You can return for multiple sessions in a single day but you don't want to overdo it. If your body is telling you to stop and you feel faint, go home and return the following day. You can always return the following day – daily sauna sessions are completely safe.

As with everything, there is a proper procedure to sweating out water weight in the sauna. First you will want to shower and dry yourself off before going into the sauna. With as little clothing as you are comfortable in, grab a towel and water and sit inside the sauna until sweat starts pouring out of your body.

To make sure your body doesn't start retaining water from dehydration, drink water at the same rate that you feel like you're losing it. As you sweat, don't be afraid to taste it to verify you are indeed sweating out the ions that are causing you to retain water.

Ions are essentially charged particles that float around in your body, having various functions. You may have heard the term "electrolyte" before. An electrolyte is a molecule with a certain electric charge in your body, such as potassium (K+), or sodium (Na+), for example.

You will want to keep sweating and drinking until you can no longer taste salt in your sweat because it is a sign that you are flushing the subcutaneous fluid and excess sodium being retained underneath the skin.

It should be noted here that while we are covering it first, utilizing the sauna for quick water weight loss is best left for last to flush the last few pounds of water. In other words, you should only use the sauna the last few days leading up to the big weigh-in or event if you have a short amount of time to drop weight. However, if you have given yourself a longer lead time, feel free to use the saunas two to three times a week in shorter intervals.

Hot Baths (Epsom Salt Bath)

While you're at the spa to use the sauna, take advantage of the hot baths or Jacuzzi tubs that are typically available to sweat out some more water. Since we sweat the most in hot, humid environments and hot water offers both heat and one hundred percent humidity, if you fully submerge everything but your nose for ten minutes at a time in the bath you will see results.

One addition you can add to your hot bath to get even better results is Epsom salt. Epsom salt is made from magnesium sulphate, which is a kind of salt that further works to suck all the moisture out of the body and reduce bloating.

Add two cups of salt in the tub and soak for about ten minutes at a time, as recommended above. As the water cools down the toxins will be sweated out of your skin.

It is important to note that regular table salt or any other type of salt cannot be substituted for the Epsom salt. Additionally, you should not take Epsom salt baths if you have heart trouble, high blood pressure or are diabetic.

Another ingredient you should consider adding to your bath is ginger. Ginger helps to open up the pores, causing you to sweat more. Add two tablespoons of grated or fresh ginger together with the two cups of Epsom salt and soak.

Finally, while taking the bath it is recommended you sip water (which can include natural or unnatural diuretics) and/or gently rub your body with a loofah or soft sponge. The loofah helps to generate more sweat. You then go to sleep without drinking, dressed warmly, and sweat out even more water.

If you do not have access to a Jacuzzi or spa you can take a hot bath at home. You want the water to be hot enough to cause moderate discomfort but not too hot so that it burns your skin. If the water in your house or apartment doesn't get that hot, you can speed the process along by heating water in kettles or pots and adding it to your bath water.

Generally hot baths or Epsom salt baths are used by fighters in ten to thirty minute sessions to dehydrate themselves one night before competition. However, you can take a bath like this every day by cutting down the length of time spent in the bath (e.g. one ten minute session), or take three to four baths per week with more sessions (e.g. two ten minute sessions) if you have a more moderate timetable to lose weight.

Body Wraps

Body wraps are another simple way to shift and remove fluid from the body. This method is known more for tightening, toning and firming up the skin, resulting in lost inches, than water weight loss on the scale. That being said, pushing fluid out from under the skin is related to water weight manipulation and I'm positive body contouring and reshaping is within the scope of interest of many of you reading this book, so I have chosen to add it to the list.

To be absolutely clear, many people who use body wraps will tout not only inches lost, but actual weight loss (from losing water weight) by employing this method. How can this be if I've just told you contouring is the main end game of wrapping? Are the people singing wrapping for weight loss wrong or am I?

Well, neither. Simply put, there are other steps typically involved in the recommended processes and procedures that accompany using body wraps, some of which we've covered, that will lead to water weight loss, but we'll get to that soon enough.

For now, suffice it to say you would be remiss to dismiss body wraps outright because results are definitely to be had (whether that be inches loss or water weight loss) and the good news is those results can last for up to three to four weeks - provided you don't undo any progress with a bad diet.

At this point, I can practically hear you shouting, "Tell me more!" To get down to brass tacks, body wraps include the use of fabric, plastic, elastic bands or garments that are wrapped around the body and left on for anywhere from forty-five minutes to eight hours (usually overnight).

The wraps themselves help to compact the soft body tissues and sculpt the body's contours. They are used in conjunction with herbal compounds, minerals and other substances, which are meant to assist in exfoliating dead skin, draw out tissue waste, and detoxify.

Sometimes the substance is separately applied to the skin prior to wrapping, and other times the wraps are soaked into a substance that has been dissolved in hot water before being applied to the client. Other times the wrap substance, such as clay, seaweed, mud or lotion, is applied directly as a wrap itself without the aid of a band or garment.

There are three basic types of body wraps commonly marketed to consumers that are supposed to target different needs and garner very specific results. All three types employ a large emphasis on moisturizing, healing and conditioning the skin, another inviting side effect for this body slimming method.

First, there are detoxifying wraps, which are designed to help cleanse the body of toxins and boost the immune system. Second, are hydrating wraps used to moisturize the skin and improve skin tone. Finally, there are inch-loss wraps that use traditional detoxifying ingredients and pressure from the way the body is wrapped to reduce fluid retention in the skin. The latter is the particular type of body wrap that we will be focusing on.

It's worth noting that all inch loss body wraps primarily work at making you appear slimmer in the same manner – and as you might have guessed it has a lot to do with fluids in the body.

Just below the skin, there are layers of fat. Within each layer of fat, there are individual fat cells, which are surrounded by interstitial fluid. This fluid can accumulate in excess within the cells and between the cells because of a lack of exercise, aging, weather, diets high in salt and sugar, Mother Nature visits and a build up of toxins.

Toxins (chemicals and preservatives) enter the body through the air we breathe, foods we eat, liquids we drink, and are absorbed through the pores in our skin from the products we apply daily to our skin and hair.

Normally, our bodies are designed to flush these toxins out through the liver and kidneys, but the amount we take in is much greater than what our bodies can safely process, so the excess toxins end up being stored in the interstitial fluid where they are then absorbed by the surrounding fat cells.

As such, some body wraps contain ingredients, such as clay, designed to absorb out these excess fluids and toxins while restoring nutrients to the body and tightening the skin.

While removing traces of toxins is a substantial component of inch loss body wraps with the proper herbs and substances, where the wraps perform a lot of their so-called magic is by compressing your skin, stimulating blood circulation and activating a process called lymphatic draining to get any remaining or excess fluid not absorbed moving along.

135

The basic way lymphatic drainage works is after plasma has delivered its nutrients and removed debris, it leaves the cells. Ninety percent of the fluid returns to the venous circulation through the venules and continues as venous blood, but 10% of this fluid becomes lymph, which is a watery fluid that contains waste products.

Unlike blood, which flows throughout the body in a continuous loop, lymph flows in only one direction within its own system – upward toward the neck. However, since the lymph doesn't have a pump like the heart, the wraps (and manual massages) aid the lymphatic system in the flowing, shifting and removal of the fluid underneath your skin.

Where does that fluid go? Well, when we move or provide pressure that is needed to encourage the flow lymph, this movement helps it filter through the lymph nodes, into the ducts, back through the blood circulatory system and into the capillaries.

Additionally, compaction squeezes the tissues together after the toxins and interstitial fluid has been extracted. Once the fluids have been extracted, there are empty pockets between the fat cells. Compressing the fat cells back together again allows for a firmer, smaller appearance.

Given the wrap's tightness and the fact that you are covered with some additional heat-generating source (plastic wrap, a thermal blanket, etc.), you will sweat out water in the localized body part resulting in temporary lost inches.

There you have it – proof body wraps can shave inches and decrease your body weight. The skeptics who claim body wraps are a scam or rip off and that they don't work at all are simply incorrect, but if you're still not convinced there is plenty of non-biased evidence on the internet of people who have posted before and after pictures or blogged about their ability to successfully trim inches and lose water weight employing this old technique.

Where the controversy and dust up comes in is when people are confused about what the wraps are actually supposed to do or how long they're supposed to do it for. As with most of the strategies in this book, body wraps won't melt your fat, burn tons of calories, or even keep your water weight loss and inches at bay forever.

The companies purposefully trying to trick consumers into believing their water weight loss, and the other techniques commonly employed with body wraps, is fat loss deserve to be raked over the coals and exposed for misleading advertising.

Any wrap company that claims their product allows you to experience weight loss by burning up to 1200 calories (as I found one unscrupulous company doing), or any other method besides the ones I've listed above is lying – plain and simple.

137

I cannot stress enough, especially since the motivation behind this book is to help those looking for the fastest way to look great by manipulating water, that any result you experience from a single wrap will be a temporary improvement. As we've already established, sometimes that's perfectly okay. By temporarily making you a little thinner so that you fit into your skinny jeans for your big reunion, you might be doubly motivated to stick to your eating and exercise plan after the reunion is said and done.

I'd also like to point out that if you continue doing the wraps on a fairly regular schedule (once or twice a week) the results are compounded and extended. You will experience long lasting tightening and toning (by long lasting, I mean as long as you keep the wrapping and everything else I've extolled - such as maintaining a good diet and moving more - constant).

However, let me posit that the advice for regular, consistent wrapping to get longer lasting, compounded effects is probably only applicable to those who are willing to make their own body wraps at home due to the costs of the other options.

If money is not an obstacle, weekly or bi-weekly wrapping can certainly be administered by professionals or by ordering / buying body wrap kits.

Let us now turn our attention to my earlier statement about the additional external processes that lend to a lot of the weight loss success associated with wraps.

If you pay close attention to the instructions doled out by wrap companies and spas you will notice almost all of them encourage the wearer to drink lots of water after administering a wrap for the effects to show up. For example, arguably one of the most popular brands/networks at the moment selling wraps direct to consumer (It Works!™ wraps) recommends drinking half your weight in ounces of water at least three days following treatment.

Just to clarify for those who are unfamiliar, resellers of this particular brand are adamant that sweating to lose water weight is not the reason their product works, and that the botanical formula on the wrap absorbed into your skin is solely responsible for the tightening and toning.

However, if you wrap something around your skin and leave it there for a period of time, no matter how you slice it, you won't be able to stop the skin underneath the wrap from sweating. It's just the way the body works.

On top of that, the resellers of this brand make it a point to stress that if you don't drink copious amounts of water in conjunction with performing the wrap it won't actually work! So in the case of this brand, what do you think is really the driving force behind your results?

Look, botanicals and herbs can be great for your skin, and I've already pointed out that you can manipulate and draw out a small amount of fluid with certain clays as well as activating lymphatic drainage, but don't fall for the okie-doke.

You are inducing sweating of the immediate area of the skin you cover with any wrap, and if you are required to drink half your body weight in water while wearing the wraps and a number of days afterwards or the product purports to not work, your weight loss (at least for that product) is primarily the result of water loss.

Drinking all of that water and running to the bathroom every thirty minutes is what truly allows your body to release pent up water being stored in the body, despite the company's claim that it's actually proof targeting water retention is definitely not a factor.

They are simply feeding off the ignorance of the general public's belief that drinking more water automatically leads to weight gain and bloat, instead of permitting your body to actually flush the water from your system.

Additionally, as a quick refresher, drinking lots of water has the other included benefits we've covered in great detail, such as making us feel fuller and less likely to consume as many calories, hydrating our bodies so everything works more harmoniously, and taking the place of the calorie laden drinks you would have ingested otherwise, such as juice or soda.

Besides promoting much higher water consumption than what most people are used to, accompanying those directions are suggestions of eating really clean, exercising and cutting back on alcohol and caffeine. Great advice, but as you well know, there's a very calculated purpose behind getting you to do these things.

It's a no brainer that if you eat really clean, exercise, and cut back on calories found in alcohol (as well as the bad dietary decisions fueled by drinking alcohol) you are bound to see some positive changes in your physique over time.

As an aside, there are other wrap companies that are upfront about the bulk of results from their wraps stemming from water weight loss. They put an emphasis on getting the skin to sweat by providing creams, pads and plastic meant to really ramp up the body temperature and shift that fluid under the skin instead of masking or being downright evasive about the way their product works.

Sure, it doesn't make other brands seem as magical as It Works!, and if there's one thing people love it's buying into miracle products that claim to be different no matter how vague or confusing the details.

However, now that you know the truth about all inch loss wraps pretty much working the same and the tricks they utilize to get enhanced results (drinking lots of water, for example) you can make an informed decision and hopefully even save money.

Finally, I would encourage you to focus on wraps that enhance the opportunity to sweat instead of trying to convince you that you are not sweating or have you sweat less. These kits will yield more drastic results than absorbent botanicals, lymph drainage and temporary displacement of fluid from the compression of the wrap alone.

The above does not mean that body wraps in and of itself is a sham or ineffective form of losing water weight, so if that's the way you find yourself feeling please go back and read the points made in the first part of this section to see why I am all in support of using this method.

It makes sense for companies to promote these additional proven techniques for fighting water retention to its customers to make their products more appealing, given the more dramatic results.

In many ways, the results that you will get purely from utilizing body wraps, without taking into consideration the add on directions to drink lots of water and eat clean, is much like what you would experience from spending time in a sweat suit (covered in more detail next), sauna or steam room.

For instance, the amount of weight that you can lose from wraps, just like saunas and sweat suits, will depend on how much excess water your body is storing right now, how hot you are able to get and the amount of time that you are able to tolerate the heat.

That being said, wraps have some differentiating factors that make them more desirable to certain people and situations. One of those factors is that body wraps provide more substantial changes in the size of certain body parts over a shorter period of time by utilizing good old compression to tighten the skin, whereas saunas and modern sweat suits by themselves do not.

So if you have a specific problem area prone to bloating and water retention or if nipping in the width of your abdomen, arms or thighs is paramount to you so that you can say - fit into a specific outfit, you might prefer wraps. The fact that you only need to focus on a specific body part at a time per session should be good news for those going the DIY route, since wrapping your whole body on your own might prove to be difficult.

It is possible to kill a few birds with one stone though when you have a few helping hands in the process, which is one of the reasons many spas offer full body wraps. Surely, the fact that the higher prices they charge needs some justification in the form of knocking as many inches off as many body parts in one shot as possible plays a part too.

When weighing the pros and cons for wraps versus the sauna, the main difference that might cause someone to prefer body wraps over the alternatives is that unlike the sauna, wraps are portable and can be applied anywhere - provided you have the scant list of materials handy.

They can be done in the privacy of your own home, which is also possible if you have an at home sauna – but most people don't, and they tend to be far cheaper and budget friendly, especially if you do them yourself.

As for how wraps stack up against sauna suits, one major difference is that wraps are disposable and cannot be reused. Another, and you might like this one, is that while sauna suits are worn in conjunction with exercise due to their generally looser fit, body wraps are typically far more restrictive when it comes to movement. Therefore, wraps are usually worn while relaxing. Nothing is stopping you from treating yourself to a wrap after a vigorous workout though!

Once you decide body wraps are something you'd like to add to your arsenal against water weight, there are tons of spas offering their services and companies that sell them catering to different price points in the marketplace. Whatever your price point, there is an option that will be right for you.

First, let's start with at home body wraps in the from of DIY kits, which can be found for anywhere from $15 to $30 plus a pop, with the variations in price boiling down to the fabric used, to the cream or which mineral and herbs the wraps were soaked in, to plain old branding and marketing (It's the same reason you pay more for Advil over a generic pharmacy brand containing the same ingredients).

Medi-spa body wrap treatments go for $50 to $100 plus depending on how many body areas are being treated. It typically involves being mummified and then hooked up to infrared machines or covered in thermal blankets and left to sweat for thirty minutes in a Zen room with a massage like atmosphere - think candles and cucumber water. Again, they have to justify the prices and create added value somehow.

Those prices are not all for naught though when you factor in overhead costs associated with having a retail space, the convenience of a technician doing all the work for you, the calming ambiance and atmosphere, and of course those huge, high tech equipment – which don't come cheap.

If you can afford and/or don't want to be bothered wrapping yourself, by all means – go to the professionals at the spa and make a day of it. You'll leave well moisturized, feeling relaxed and pampered, and if done right, your clothes fitting a little looser than when you walked in.

By the way do not underestimate the power of relaxing and de-stressing for weight loss purposes. When you get stressed out your cortisol levels increase, and that's bad because your appetite is increased. If you've ever turned to food while undergoing a stressful period of your life, cortisol is partly to thank, or blame.

Cortisol stimulates fat and carbohydrate metabolism for fast energy, and stimulates insulin release and maintenance of blood sugar levels. Additionally, studies have shown links to higher cortisol and higher belly fat.

Now, for those of you who already have a de-stressing ritual in place, might be bothered by the up-close and personal attention from a perfect stranger, or would rather not - or frankly cannot - drop the kind of coin involved to have name brand wraps delivered via subscription to your home or luxurious spa treatments replete with special mystery detoxifying clay every week, there's hope for you yet.

I'm happy to report you can still experience the shrinking and tightening benefits from wrapping by making your own at home body wrap. Doing so is surprisingly easy and affordable to boot.

To prepare your skin for the wrap, if possible, start by taking a warm shower to open your pores up and allow quick absorption of the minerals. To aid in this objective, you will want to exfoliate with a sugar or salt scrub or another exfoliator that will not leave a residue while showering.

Don't have an expensive scrub on hand? No worries – here's a very simple recipe that can be used for this first step in the process: you will need coconut, olive or canola oil, sugar or sea salt. Optional items such as a loofah exfoliation sponge, mitt or brush, and essential oils such as tea tree oil or lavender oil for fragrance, will make the exfoliating process easier and more relaxing.

Mix one part oil and two parts sugar or salt - adjusted to suit your personal needs (e.g. 1 tablespoon or oil to 2 tablespoons of sugar or salt), along with two drops of your essential oil together. Then using the loofah, mitt, brush or your hands, apply a generous amount all over your body. Rinse thoroughly to cleanse the skin and then dry yourself off with a clean towel.

Do not moisturize with any of your regular lotions or creams prior to the wrap. Again, the point of the above scrub is to remove any pore clogging ingredients so your skin is left clean and open to be ready for the body wrap solution. Commercial brand lotions and creams will result in clogged pores and decrease your ability to absorb your wrap solution and/or sweat more.

The next step after your cleansing shower won't be the same for everyone. It will be dependent on your personal preference, time constraints and the collection of supplies you are able to gather, as there are a couple of variations to the order of events in body wrapping.

Before I get into the options you have available to you, just so you know the general order of things, the second step consists of applying the oils/compounds and wrapping yourself. To do that, you'll need to gather some integral ingredients and supplies.

First – quite obviously, you will need some type of bandage. Ace bandages are a cheap fan favorite among body wrap Do-It-Yourselfers, and can be found at your local pharmacy or dollar store. When selecting which type of bandage, I suggest you steer clear of the self-adhesive bandages, as they can cause skin tears, and opt for the ones with metal clips.

Don't feel like spending money on strips of bandages or making a trip to the store? That's fine - you can improvise and use a piece of fabric from an old article of clothing or a cotton sheet cut in nice long strips if you want. If you have any sewing skills reposition a button or two and their accompanying slits to make for a tight hold in place of the clips found on the Ace bandages.

Other items you will want to gather include a quality plastic wrap such as saran wrap or cling wrap, a heating source such as a heated blanket or hot water bottle/pad (not required but highly recommended), a small bowl for mixing ingredients, and the ingredients themselves to make your very own toxin and fluid ridding solution the spas and wrap companies love boasting about.

Personally, I like to use a mixture of sea salt or Epsom salt, coconut oil, and other organic ingredients such as organic caffeinated green tea bags to stimulate circulation, herbal extracts to draw out accumulated toxins that sit on the skin and soft tissue layers, and essential oils.

When it comes to making your own, you can copy my preferred mixture to the tee, or you can draw inspiration from my mix and modify things to your liking. You can also go rogue and do your own thing entirely with the plethora of compounds and options for pairing them together out there.

To help you in that process, I have taken the liberty of providing a detailed list of some of the most common ingredients added to the solution base, and how they benefit your skin below. Again, the possibilities are nearly endless, so I would recommend buying what you can obtain easily and fits into your budget.

Once you have everything ready boil 1.8lts of water in a large stainless steel pot. Once it has reached boiling point remove it from the heat and add all your selected ingredients and allow it to cool down for 10 minutes before using it.

Clays

Dead Sea - Mineral and nutrient enriched for detoxification

Earth - Oily skin, exfoliates and stimulates circulation

Green Clay – Detoxifies, oily skin, stimulates circulation

Moroccan Red – Exfoliates, stimulates circulation Fullers

Natural Clay: Choose 2 cups of clay suitable for your skin type.

Red Clay -Stimulated circulation, removes dry skin cells

Rose Clay -Exfoliates, stimulates circulation

Salt: (Choose 1 cup of salt)

Dead Sea Salt -Skin tonic, detoxifying, nutrient enriched

Epsom Salts – Relaxes the nervous system eases pain and

removes toxins

Sea Salt - Draws toxins from the body

Herbs: (1 cup in total)

Alfalfa Leaf powder – Relives muscle and joint pain, fatigue

Aloe Vera – Soothes and Heals

Calendula powder - Heals broken skin

Chamomile Powder – Anti inflammatory, Calming

Kelp Powder: (1 cup) To detoxify the body and add vital nutrients that help reduce cellulite and increase circulation

Neem Leaves – Anti bacterial, anti fungal

Parsley Powder - Detoxifying, soothing

Peppermint Leaf – Stimulation, soothing, stomach upset

Rose Petal Powder – Stimulates Circulation

Rosehip Powder - Vitamin c, nutrients

St Johns Wart Powder – Healing nutrient

Stinging Nettles Powder - Deep cleanser, soothes irritated skin

Moisture Agents: (Substitute any of these agents for water)

Apple Cider Vinegar – Helps to heal bruises, soothes irritated skin

Chamomile - Promotes relaxation and detoxifies

Fruit Juice – Full of vitamins

Glycerin – Deep skin Moisturizer

Goats Milk - Balances PH levels in skin and exfoliates skin cells whilst moisturizing

Lemon Juice – detoxifies and cleanses skin cells

Whole Cream Milk - Relieves dry and itchy skin and full of nutrients

Witch Hazel - Skin toner and cleanser

Yogurt - Soothes dry and irritated skin

Essential Oils - 18mls in total combined oils Or 1% of mix These essential oils are used to combat cellulite and detoxify the body

Basil Essential Oil- Anti bacterial, headaches, mental alertness, fatigue, stress, and period pains.

Cypress Essential Oil- Diuretic, varicose veins, circulation, coughs and colds.

Fennel Essential Oil – Diuretic, circulation. Cleansing oil, indigestion and gas.

Juniper Berry Essential Oil -Cellulite, uplifting

Lavender Essential Oil – Headaches, stress, insomnia, minor burns, skin rashes, lowers blood pressure. Calmative.

Lemon Essential Oil- Cellulite, oily skin, anti bacterial, asthma and other respiratory complaints.

Lemon Grass Essential Oil – Skin toner, oily skin, fatigue, muscle aches and gastric infections.

Patchouli Essential Oil – Tightens pores, combats wrinkles, Mobilizes cellulite, stress reliever, insomnia, relaxant, acne, eczema, psoriasis, sores and minor burns

Sandalwood Essential Oil- Calms the mind and spirit, oily skin, soothes irritated skin, and is an aphrodisiac for men.

Spearmint Essential Oil – Soothes the skin, calmative, and settles upset tummies.

Tea Tree Essential Oil – Anti- fungal, acne, skin toner.

Natural Additives: (2 tablespoons of any)

Aloe Vera Gel - moisturizer Rice Bran Powder Fine- Prevents

wrinkles, exfoliates skin, absorbs excess oil and dirt

Honey Powder- Skin cleaners, softener, absorbs dry skin.

Coconut Milk Powder - Skin softener, full of nutrients

Moisturizing Oils: (2 tablespoons in total only)

Almond Oil - mature skin, sensitive or dry skin

Aloe Vera Oil – anti-ageing, skin irritations, cuts and minor burns

Apricot Kernel Oil- Skin irritations, dry inflamed skin. Absorbs quickly.

Evening primrose Oil- eczema, nourishes dry skin

Flaxseed Oil – eczema, psoriasis, acne and aging skin

Macadamia Oil- Penetrates the skin quickly, anti oxidant

Olive Oil- regenerate new skin cells, draws moisture to external skin cells

Palm Oil – Moisturizing oil

Rapeseed Oil - strengths skin tissue full of vitamins and minerals

Refined Emu Oil- repairs damaged and wrinkled skin, muscle and joint pain, repairs scar tissue.

Sesame Oil- moisturizing, retains skins elasticity

Shea Oil – retains skins elasticity, moisturizes dry cracked skin

Soybean Oil- moisturizing oil filled with vitamin E

Sunflower Oil- moisturizes, regenerate and condition skin

Of course, while some people love all aspects of the do-it-yourself approach to body wraps, others prefer the convenience of leaving certain elements (such as mixing solutions) to the pros.

This makes perfect sense since the appeal of doing a wrap yourself probably has a lot to do with saving money and time, so the thought of having to put a lot of both into tracking down and purchasing the aforementioned individual ingredients, then mixing them together might turn you right off wraps altogether.

For those of you who fit into this category, buying something pre-made that already incorporates most of the essential ingredients you desire is your best bet. However, if you go this route, be careful to read all the ingredients to avoid putting harmful stabilizers and compounds typically found in big batch products on your skin.

If you're looking for a specific product recommendation, the only product I can personally vouch for is my own, which is made up of only the most effective, highest quality ingredients and available for sale in my Etsy shop, http://www.etsy.com/thighgaphack.

Many of my solutions contain the items on the list and you will not have to buy anything additional. Please note, I am offering 15% off items for my readers using the code ETSYTGH. I will gladly answer any questions you have and can alter any recipe to be used for the slimming wrap.

Now that you have your solution in place, you have two ways in which to apply it. Option number one is reminiscent of the home wrapping kits that you would buy from a company like It Works!

Heat the solution to 120 degrees F in a heating unit (pot on the stove top, slow cooker, crock pot, etc.). Soak your bandages or pieces of cloth in the solution for 30 minutes to allow the solution to be absorbed into the wraps.

Allow the solution to cool to a temperature that is still hot but tolerable to the touch. Use tongs to remove the wraps from the heated solution one at a time as needed. Wear gloves to wring out the excess water from the wrap prior to wrapping. Follow up with saran wrap before securing with a girdle or other fabric to keep the plastic in place.

Option number two is to apply a thin layer of the solution to the skin first *then* wrap the area in saran wrap, followed up by a bandage to keep the plastic in place. Instead of a bandage, some people opt for a girdle or shape wear, which serves the same purpose.

In this version, applying the saran wrap directly to the skin works to lock in your body heat and prevent you from cooling down, thus forcing your sweat glands to work overtime, as opposed to relying as heavily on the creams/concoctions to do the job of pulling out fluid. Therefore, you might choose to go this route if you don't have a solution or lots of ingredients in your solution.

The logical question you may be asking yourself at this point is, which way is better? Neither is right or wrong, just different with pros and cons that will or will not fit your personal preference.

For example, many prefer the second method because it is faster, requires fewer products and supplies, is less messy, as you are not soaking the fabric and dealing with drip drops everywhere, and you can re-use the ace bandages.

However, to get the best results using the second or "dry" method, you will need to help generate as much heat as possible by doing light house work, going for a walk or out and about while wearing the wrap.

Conversely, using the wet or first method relies more heavily on the herbs/creams to moisturize and detoxify the skin so you get two forces combating your fluid retention as opposed to one. Your skin may also feel smoother and softer as a result of this method.

Once you figure out which method to use, your next hurdle will be mastering the art of wrapping. Remember, while you want to wrap tight please be careful not to wrap to the point where you cannot breath. This can cause severe circulatory problems.

The tricky part for many people is getting the plastic to cooperate without slipping. A handy plastic wrap dispenser like the ones that furniture movers use, or keeping the plastic taught on the roll instead of pre-tearing pieces) really works best.

A good technique is to overlap the wraps, making sure the lower edges cross the middle of the previous wrap. To secure each wrap firmly, twist the end and tuck into the previous wrap. This will allow you to wrap the plastic fairly tightly on your limbs and torso and get out of the wrap safely and effectively.

You can easily place the wrap on yourself in most cases, especially if you are doing one body part, but occasionally you may come across areas that might require some help, such as the arms. Either recruit a friend or family member to help or do one side at a time.

The final last step (again, optional but recommended) is to cover yourself with a warm blanket or heating pad. Stay wrapped up and warm and cozy for at least half an hour. This will help make the treatment more effective.

To wrap things up (pun intended), before you run out and gather your supplies or order my scrub on Etsy, I'd like to leave you with some words of wisdom and cautions to consider in order to ascertain whether body wraps might be a good fit for you.

If you have sensitive skin, beware of body wrap ingredients that have a lot of fragrance. They could irritate your skin. This is not so much of an issue when mixing up your own concoctions in your living room as when purchasing pre-made wraps or getting one done at a spa. Be sure to ask about or read over the list of ingredients before choosing a wrap. Generally, clay is less irritating to the skin than fragrant oils.

It's also important to find out the ingredients of a body wrap beforehand if you are taking any prescription medications. Then, call your doctor to see if there are any problems. Herbals can be absorbed through the skin and potentially alter the effectiveness of some medications.

Also, you might want to at least give a few seconds of thought towards whether or not you can comfortably tolerate wrapping. If you are claustrophobic or have issues with being wrapped like a mummy, or having restricted movement of your limbs, body wraps are probably not the best option for you. You'd be better off utilizing the sauna or sweat suit.

In the same vein, it it can be embarrassing or uncomfortable to some to have another person wrapping your body in plastic or applying exfoliating and moisturizing products to intimate regions. Mull over this fact before deciding to pay a visit to the spa to get the service performed.

The boilerplate disclaimer applies; Body wraps should never be used by women who are pregnant, breast-feeding, those who are taking medications that make them susceptible to heat, or anyone who is suffering from existing health conditions. Body wraps can be uncomfortable for some people, though the results can often be worth it. Lastly, don't forget to stay hydrated to replenish the water in your body and prevent dehydration.

Sweat Suits

Sweat suits, also known as rubber suits because the first variations were made of rubberized cloth, sauna suits, and in some instances otherwise used as garbage bags, are made from waterproof material and are designed so that the body retains heat and moisture causing the wearer to sweat profusely.

As previously mentioned there are only four ways to actually get the water out of your body - urine, sweat, feces, and respiration, or the air you exhale. Not surprisingly, sauna suits contribute to weight loss by inducing sweating and interfering with the body's cooling system.

You see the body functions at its best at an internal temperature of approximately 98.6 degrees and works hard to maintain this temperature. When our body temperature rises above this, there are several cooling systems in place, the most significant of which is sweat or more precisely, the evaporation of sweat.

Sweat rate varies depending on many factors including the internal production of heat, the environmental temperature, humidity, the type of clothing worn, as well as others. Exercise raises the internal production of heat so our sweating rate increases in order to help cool the body.

When a sauna suit is worn, however, the sweat cannot evaporate thanks in part to the material (typically pvc, vinyl, tyvek or coated nylon cloth) and the construction of the suits – closures at the waist, neck, wrists, and ankles are all elasticated to help retain body heat and moisture within the garment, with some including hoods to provide additional retention of body heat; therefore cooling does not take place and you keep sweating away.

This leads to an even greater rise in body temperature and even more sweating as the body continues to attempt to cool itself down. Thus, the cycle continues — further rise in temperature, more sweating, further rise in temperature, more sweating, ad infinitum.

A significant amount of fluid is lost and results in you looking slimmer and trimmer. You can lose up to five pounds in one session and while many believe the water weight will return the second you bring a glass of water or fluid to your lips, making sauna suits worthless or the time spent sweating all for naught, you can indeed reap the results for longer than a 24-hour period.

The water weight lost from sweating will not just come back immediately. The American College of Sports Medicine reports that it may take up to 72 hours to replenish glycogen and fluid balance. So for the purposes of looking great for an event or cutting weight for a weigh in, sauna suits are perfectly fine. If you rotate your suit every three or so days and incorporate all the other dietary tips in this book to fend off water retention the cumulative effects will be noticeable and long lasting.

Having said that, now would be a great opportunity to stress the importance of drinking water before, during and after using the sauna suits, precisely because you don't have to fear doing so will immediately cancel out all of your efforts.

It may seem counterintuitive, but drinking water before, during and after your session serves to prevent dehydration and coax the body to get rid of the retained water. Plus, you now know you have at least three days before all that new water you've ingested might show up on the scale (if you fail to incorporate the other advice within these pages).

Another reason sauna suits aren't meaningless is because elevating your body temperature slightly increases your metabolic rate while you work out in your suit due to the additional work of ventilation (breathing rate), enzyme activity and increase in sweat gland activity. Research gives a figure of 4% to 10% increase of metabolic heat release (measured in calories) on average. While that may not be astronomical it is far better than a big fat goose egg.

This increase will last a short time after you stop wearing the sweat suit and working out (about thirty minutes to an hour). So while it's not remotely doing the entire calorie burning work for you, the suit does make a contribution towards your goal of losing weight with the combined water weight loss and higher metabolism, which you would not have gotten otherwise without it.

Besides the obvious aforementioned effects, some of the other benefits for choosing sauna sweat suits are: they provide an inexpensive and time saving alternative to a real sauna with costs range from as little as $13 to upwards of $80 or more. The difference in price can be attributed to the make and feel of the suit but at such a large price range a sweat suit is accessible to just about anyone.

The suits are lightweight and portable so you can bring it with you while traveling on vacation or business trips and are also comfortable enough to wear during your daily workout regimen or just around the home. They are ideal for keeping muscles warm and relaxed, and are effective at getting toxins and impurities out of your body and skin.

Sauna suits are commonly worn under or over jogging clothes during physical exercise (newer suits boast updated, modern designs so that they no longer look conspicuously out of place and so can be worn without other noticing in public), but they can also be worn alone for body wrapping in some health spas. There are also creams that can be purchased for use under the suit to further induce sweating.

Alternatives to full body suits, like a slimmer belt, which is a form-fitting neoprene belt worn around the waist to promote sweating, and sauna shorts, which are designed to be worn under clothing as you work out, may also be considered.

Whatever you choose to buy, be sure they will hold up under the stress of whatever activity you will be participating in. On that subject, any and every activity is not equally suited – please excuse the pun - for performing in a sauna suit.

For example, you should not be doing three-hour long treadmill stints, and intense heavy resistance training workouts or lifting sessions; otherwise be prepared to become dizzy and pass out. This is because your body's ability to perform at a *high* level during exercise is actually diminished from the core-heating effect that sauna suits cause. This is also precisely why sauna suits are best used as a temporary solution for tackling water weight loss and not fat loss, as the title of this book suggests.

The exercise that compliments sauna suits best is low to moderate intensity steady state cardio for thirty minutes to sixty minutes maximum. Longer time frames (a few hours) are permissible if just sitting or working around the house in them. They are not intended for use while sleeping, as it's too dangerous to wear that long without monitoring how much water weight you've lost, and they should absolutely not be worn in a sauna.

Because sauna suits work amazingly well at doing what they promise to do (make you sweat) you must be careful and smart when incorporating it into your weight loss plan, as there are dangers and risks involved with improper use. For example, wearing a sauna suit while working out in high temperature climates could lead to overheating or heat stroke, extreme loss of electrolytes, dehydration, loss of consciousness, cardiovascular related emergencies, and in the most extreme and reckless cases, death.

As with all things, start using your sauna suit in moderation, especially until you get used to it. Three to four times a week is a good place to start, and definitely no more than once a day. After a period of time you should stop and give your body a rest, as these suits should only be incorporated short tem and not on an ongoing basis.

A good time frame to work within is two to three weeks of intermittent use before taking at least as long of a time period (two to four weeks off) without the suits. Remember, the fact of the matter is you are tampering with the body's functions – ability to cool down, heat regulation, etc. and if you do this long term it could take years for your body to reestablish normality.

The goal is to utilize this tool without reaching the point of diminishing returns. I know, it may seem tempting to up the frequency or length of time to get faster results, but sometimes more is not always better, so please take heed of my advice.

On top of exercising moderation you should always listen to your body while wearing the sweat suit and use common sense to avoid compromising your overall health. If you feel you're getting too overheated, by all means, remove the suit, get cooler, and drink plenty of rehydrating liquids.

Compression Garments

Compression garments are making a huge comeback these days, but we now call them body shapers. Your spanxx, waist trainers, girdles, corsets, etc. are all modern day compression garments.

You can do your part to increase your inch loss results and maintain your new shape even longer by purchasing a body shaper and wearing that each day for about a week after your wrap. As your body continues to eliminate toxins as natural waste material (you are drinking more water!), you will notice additional inch loss and body toning if you wear a firm body shaper. These do not have to be expensive. For a woman, one that goes from mid-calf to just under the breasts is best. For a man, a body shaper with firm support through the stomach and upper thighs is best. These are not to be worn at night.

Laxatives

Highly controversial and largely frowned upon because of its potentially harmful effects, laxatives in and of itself is just another tool in your toolshed that can be used to move water weight. They are relatively inexpensive and the fact of the matter is in the short term, can be safe and effective at slimming you down. The way you use or abuse them is what makes laxatives good or bad.

First and foremost, laxatives work by stimulating the colon and large intestine to expel the contents. In other words, the laxatives help you digest your food a little faster than normal, flushes out what is left in your stomach and then goes through the intestines and gets the left overs. This does not mean your entire lower intestine will be emptied but generally it will be cleaned out enough to see a difference on the scale and flatten a protruding belly.

Their primary use is for those who have constipation, which is a symptom where one gets dry stool and the evacuation is difficult and infrequent, and are very bloated and blocked up from not expelling waste on a regular basis. Of course, there are other natural ways to relieve constipation, such as drinking lots of water before and after meals and adding more fiber rich foods to your diet to your diet to help speed up bowel movement.

However, any adult can obtain and take the anti-constipation medication and many do. In fact, a recent study showed that the United Sates has the highest rate of laxative use compared to several other countries[3], and a separate study gave a more in depth perspective on the prevalence of laxative use by providing a monetary figure to the industry in the amount of $700 million spent each year.

Additionally, in a 2013 poll conducted by online pharmacy UKMedix.com, more than half of women dieters admitted to using laxatives for a quick fix, as it causes rapid weight and water loss from the body.[4]

What are the chances that despite those high figure of laxative usage, which might I add, topped fasting and sweat suits in the list of weight loss techniques polled, the majority of dieters who have tried laxatives are not walking around addicted or abusing them? My guess is really high.

You see, despite the fear mongering of the media that would have you believe taking one or a few laxatives as a dieting aid to quickly shed unwanted weight for a special occasion automatically means you're done in for, in reality that is not really the case.

---

[3] Denisko, Yelena. "Laxatives: Proceed with Caution." Web blog post. Consumer Health Information Corporation. 2011.

[4] Harding, Eleanor. "Half of Women Dieters Admit Using Laxatives for Quick-fix Weight Loss at Least once Despite knowing it's Bad for Their Health." Web blog post. Daily Mail. Associated Newspapers Ltd. 01 October 2013. Web. 01 October 2013.

Hundreds of thousands of mentally sound and reasonable people manage to use laxatives safely as intended and for its off label use (any use not included in the FDA regulations) of dropping water weight. The problem occurs when those with misunderstandings of what laxatives can do and mental illnesses or susceptibility to mental disorders get their hands on the medication.

As such, it is worth stressing the fact that fat loss does not enter the picture since by the time food gets into the large intestine everything has been absorbed by the upper digestive tract (i.e. – the stomach and small intestine). So, if you have consumed more calories than you were supposed to in a given day there's no reversing that regardless of how many laxatives you take.

Yes, the expelling of the contents from the bowels will result in weight loss on the scale, and for many people, a flatter tummy, but it is strictly from water/fluid being lost, and going back to an earlier metaphor, the emptying of the rocks in your pocket.

Hopefully, I have cleared up some of the misconceptions, both good and bad, surrounding the use of laxatives, and can now move on to the best and safest way to utilize them for your purposes. First, you should know that not all laxatives are created equal. There are four types that range in intensity:

Laxative Type #1: The least powerful laxative is a fiber-based laxative that bulks up the stool and helps it pass naturally through the digestive system.

Laxative Type #2: The next laxative type that is a little stronger are the osmotic laxatives that work by drawing water into the intestine and helps the stool move through quicker.

Laxative Type #3: A stronger laxative type is the stool softeners that make the stool soft and is used for people who are constipated and having difficult bowel movements.

Laxative Type #4: The strongest laxative type is the stimulant laxatives that actually irritate the intestinal walls forcing the body to expel whatever is in the digestive tract.

Given the options, by far the safest types of laxatives to use are mild and natural bulk laxatives, such as psyllium (Metamucil) and methylcellulose (Citrucel). They make the stool more bulky by absorbing water. For example, psyllium (Metamucil) is safe because it is a natural form of fiber.

In contrast, Laxatives that quickly produce a bowel movement, such as Senna (Senokot) or bisacodyl (Dulcolax), tend to be the most abused and dangerous. They stimulate the nerves in the colon, causing the muscles of the intestines to contract and push down the contents of the bowel.

Again, this doesn't mean that you cannot use these products without automatically abusing them or putting your body in danger. It simply means if you opt for the stronger and more fast acting laxatives, you can only use them very sparingly and as a last minute boost – e.g. a day or two before your event.

Otherwise, regular prolonged use over time will result in keeping the colon empty, and inhibit it from sending the signal for a normal bowel movement to occur. It continues to go downhill from there as the muscles of the bowel become weakened because they are not being used, and the body gradually gets used to needing laxatives to produce a bowel movement. This can occur in as little as a week.

Ignorance of the serious side effects of aggressive laxatives like the aforementioned is one of the primary reasons people ignore the important parameters to their peril and end up spiraling out of control. You see, where a lot of people go wrong – and what a lot of health experts should focus their criticism on instead of proclaiming all laxatives as bad – is overdoing laxatives by either taking them too long and/or taking too many at a given time (overdosing).

I believe if the entire picture is presented and people are informed of the benefits and consequences of misuse of laxatives, they would make better decisions and plan to incorporate laxatives without going down the slippery slope of addiction.

I believe this because I've heard from people who abused laxatives that they had no idea that they couldn't lose calories from using laxatives or had no idea of the negative long-term effects when they started using them. They go on to state that had they known they would have never made the decisions they had – like taking 20 to 30 pills a day or using it daily.

With that said, although listed here as a viable option for losing water weight loss I cannot stress enough that the danger of laxatives is very real and occurs from chronic over use and abuse (taking them every day over a long period of time or while fasting).

The reason is you lose most of the bacteria you need for normal digestion and since you also lose electrolytes, the imbalance can cause you to feel dizzy and/or pass out. Additionally, if you take laxatives long enough they can cause constipation, problems with your sphincters, and as I alluded to earlier, eventually even stop working.

This is why it is so important to use this tool in a smart and responsible way. This means not using laxatives as a way to binge or eat crappy food under the erroneous mindset that everything that you eat will be washed away magically. It also means remaining hydrated and taking supplements like calcium that will restore important anti-oxidants to the body.

When it comes to this stuff, more is not better, that is unless you like experiencing nasty and painful side effects. For this method, the minimum effective dose really comes into play. For those who are unfamiliar with this term, the minimum effective dose is the idea that doing something beyond a certain point is wasteful and inefficient.

For example, if water boils at 212 degrees Fahrenheit (100 degrees Celsius), heating up water to anything above 212 degrees Fahrenheit when your objective is to boil water is wasted energy. Why spend unnecessary time waiting an extra few minutes to get that water temperature to 300 degrees when the job was done at 212?

With laxatives, the same holds true. To lose water weight with this method, you want to take the least amount of laxatives necessary to trigger the processes in the body. Since every brand and type will differ, refer to the recommended dosage listed on the package (don't go more than one pill over) and perhaps even start by taking half of the recommended dose. Also be sure to not exceed the time frame written on the package.

Generally, you should plan to take the recommended amounts on the box before your largest meal for no more than one to two weeks (or shorter if directed by the brand). If doing two weeks, you may want to break things up by taking the laxatives two to three nights apart (do not take daily in any instance). As you can see, there is no mistaking this method of weight loss as anything but a very short-term solution.

Anything more and you are simply wasting pills, risking addiction or dependency on them, creating an environment for your body to become immune to the effects and possibly endangering your health.

Meanwhile it is imperative to drink plenty of water as you can become dehydrated. This combination should give you the results you seek with minimal to no cramping and allow for your body to go back to a normal regularity.

Note that if you are drinking plenty of water and following the diet portion of this book you should have no problem going to the bathroom every day.

If you don't heed my advice get ready to feel like death warmed over. I'm not kidding folks - the nausea, painful cramps, dizziness and hot and cold flashes people report are not pretty. On top of that, being unable to go to the bathroom naturally anymore and experiencing constant bowl blockages is not fun.

Since ingesting laxatives will have the inconvenient side effect of sending you to the rest room on a regular basis, timing is key. When you choose to take them needs to be carefully orchestrated taking your schedule into careful consideration.

The best time to take laxatives for most people will be around mid morning or mid day so that they take effect part way through the night. Taking them at night will definitely send you to the bathroom in the morning and might not stop until mid morning, which won't be ideal if you have to go to work or school.

One thing to be aware of before going the laxative route is if you are on any sort of medication currently, laxatives can actually make your medication less effective. In many cases they can actually remove any effect your medication is supposed to have for you so check with your doctor or abstain from use altogether if you are unsure of its effects on your medication.

Finally, as with everything in life, there is more than one way to skin a cat. For those of you naturalists, there are other natural options besides artificial stimulants that work much like laxatives that you would purchase in your pharmacy. For example, drinking salt water, black current tea, milk of magnesia, taking magnesium citrate, castor oil or filling up on fiber has a similar effect on the body. You can also take a pure veggie laxative, which is a little more expensive, but is like taking concentrated prunes.

Many of these alternatives are stimulant free and thus will not cause cramping, but that doesn't mean that you have free reign to abuse these substances either. They should be treated just as the laxatives in pill form and used sparingly for only a short time.

Enema

Enemas are an important treatment for constipation usually associated with the cleaning of the colon and have been around since the dawn of time, so if you elect to participate in this method you will be in good company.

To give you a more specific idea of that company – Ancient regions in Africa, Greece, Babylonia, India and China used enemas; American Indians were known to use enemas; Louis XIV had almost two thousand enemas in his lifetime and stayed healthy throughout; The vivacious and voluptuous Mae West reportedly started every day with a morning enema, and even biblical scripts have shown recorded use.

You see, before the widespread use of IV's and Nasogastric tubes as a method of administering medicine and nutrients, the enema was a very widely used method to administer pain medications, alleviate certain conditions or to nourish and hydrate the patient.

However, since every thing old is not automatically good (although there is no debating the fact that we are standing on the shoulders of giants who were brilliant thinkers in the past), it is important to note that enemas are still used today by holistic physicians for all sorts of conditions including cancer.

They are frequently used in natural cancer protocol such as the Gerson Therapy and were outlined as a treatment in the revered "Merck Manul", a book used by physicians as their primary reference for decades.

Given the fact that enemas have been around the block more than a few times, there have been numerous studies and anecdotes given on their purported benefits. Just a few of the reported positive results include relaxation, a better mood, more energy, refreshing sleep, help with fatigue, liver detoxification, greater mental clarity and last but not least – water weight loss.

Actually, for most people who perform enemas weight loss is not the primary goal, but when you consider that the average person may have up to ten pounds or more of non-eliminated waste in the large intestine, using an enema to flush waste out of the colon to exclusively drop pounds doesn't seem like such an absurd idea. Of course, the additional benefits listed above are like icing on the cake.

As you may have gathered, an enema works as a weight loss tool as a bowel stimulant, similar to a laxative. The main difference is that laxatives are commonly thought of as orally administered while enemas are administered directly into the rectum, and thereafter, into the colon. Enemas also instantly leave you feeling cleaner, lighter and healthier and doesn't drag on for as long as the results of a laxative – a plus in most people's book.

The way enemas are performed is very straightforward, albeit not for the faint hearted. Essentially, liquids are injected into the rectum through the help of specific equipment in order to relieve the body of waste. Warm water is usually used in order to perform the task, however other liquids including herbal tea, coffee, or water mixed with salt might also be used.

Caffeine is particularly popular amongst the enema practicing crowd as it is an ergogenic aid, a stimulant and an appetite suppressant, so it might make it easier for you to exercise, force you to exercise, and help you eat less.

The cost of an enema ranges widely. You can pay $100 or more for a boutique enema where a through cleansing is performed by a specialist with the help of equipment specifically designed for this purpose. You can also perform enemas from the comfort of your own home, which can be an inexpensive option – especially if you order all of your materials, like the coffee (optional), an enema bag, hooks, tubing, oil, and pipes separately.

Note that I said doing an at home enema *can be* an inexpensive option instead of making an absolute statement about it being so, because you can end up spending just as much money initially, if not more, with a DIY option. For example, a full home kit with everything you need already included can be purchased at a drug store or the Internet for anywhere from $20 for the disposable options to $150 or more.

It should be pointed out though that while the more pricey kits are comparable to the cost of having one boutique enema, the higher upfront investment for the at home option is typically spread over multiple enemas thus being cost effective and a more attractive option to regular users.

That being said, if you know you are particularly squeamish or only plan on utilizing an enema once or twice to help meet your weight loss goal, you may want to forget about DIY and research a specialist in your area to do the treatment for you.

For the rest of you fearless enough to take matters into your own hands, the question you might be asking yourself is if there is a real benefit for the more expensive kits or if shelling out lots of dough for fancier tubes will be in vain?

To answer your question, generally spending more money on a kit is warranted as the differences in price can be attributed to variables such as the brand name, quality, design and sophistication of the materials.

For example, stainless steel enema buckets and silicone enema bags with silicone hosing are the least toxic set-ups available and therefore more expensive. If you can afford it, it is worth the extra money, as they will minimize the leaching of toxins into the enema.

On the other hand, latex and soft plastic (vinyl and otherwise) or disposable plastic enema kits are cheaper because the lower grade material is intended for single use and the ability to prevent leaching is diminished. As such, they are not as recommended, except perhaps occasionally while traveling and pressed for time. The environmental impact of disposable kits (if that matters to you) is yet another reason to invest in a more expensive reusable kit.

Keep in mind that whatever material you use for a container, you should minimize the time the coffee sits in it to minimize leaching of toxins into the coffee, tea or water, and make sure to thoroughly clean the equipment before and after each use.

One of the reasons enemas have stood the test of time is complications as a result of performing enemas are highly unusual. That being said, by no means are enemas 100% side effect free. Just as with any treatment, it is not without its fair share of risks if used improperly.

Those risks include perforation of the rectum, which requires surgery to repair and possible damage to internal organs, and septicemia - otherwise known as bacteria in the bloodstream. Furthermore, the "washing" out of the rectum and intestine can interfere with your body's normal absorption of nutrients and fluids, leading to chemical imbalances.

Also, much like laxatives, people can develop a dependency if they make a habit of using enemas to create bowel movements, and may experience electrolyte imbalances in the body called hyponatremia, in which the blood becomes diluted and its salt content becomes lower than normal.

These are all valid concerns and throughout the process of using enemas, we must continually try to avoid danger and maximize benefits by exercising moderation and adhering to the safety rules before attempting an enema.

Doing so is most definitely in your best interest because you do not want to deal with any of the above issues *on top* of trying to lose weight. Speaking of moderation, perhaps the most important place to start is with how often is too often to turn to enemas for weight loss.

The daily enema of kings and celebrities notwithstanding, the magic number necessary and recommended to lose weight is nowhere near that amount. In fact, it should be stressed that using enemas to lose weight are on a separate playing field than using them to combat physical maladies. While some people commit daily enemas when trying to heal an ailment, two to three times a week is generally the maximum recommended amount for our purposes.

Another factor to consider in the quest for the optimal recommended amount is the type of enema you choose to do. As long as you are doing plain water enemas you can perform them whenever you feel backed up for up to a week before taking a break to allow the microbes to repopulate.

Stronger enemas, such as coffee enemas, should be done a lot more infrequently. Experts recommend once every few weeks or a more conservative once a month. As most of you will be trying to lose weight in a short time period, which means you'll only be able to complete one or two before your special occasion or weigh in.

That being said, you might want to save this type of enema for two to three days before as a last minute boost in achieving your goal weight/physique.

The second most important set of guidelines you need to adhere to if you want to avoid negative side effects involve the proper administration of an enema. Going rogue or taking bad advice could end very badly so it is imperative you thoroughly read and adhere to the steps outlined below.

Please note, while this section may seem to only be geared towards those who plan on doing a DIY enema, even if you go to a specialist at a seemingly reputable place to get one done, the following will help you know exactly what to expect and what to question or be wary of while under someone else's care.

Keep in mind everyone offering such services will not be equally competent or as diligent as they should be. Some people will cut corners to save money or put you in danger with an overly rigorous approach. There are as many different claims for how to best administer an enema as there are petals on a daisy, and all you need to do is unwittingly choose the wrong person and allow yourself to be mishandled to pay the ultimate price. Ignorance is not bliss.

The following is a list of the specific ingredients, equipment and necessities that are par for the course with the treatment: an enema bag or bucket (buckets are easier to clean and dry while bags allow you to control the flow more easily and observe the flow of the enema), lubricant or any edible oil, something to hang the bag on if self administered, a good location (the bed or in the bathroom either lying on a rug or in the bathtub), a pad or old heavy bath towel to be placed under you during the enema.

A water enema will require about two quarts (about eight cups), but no more than three quarts of purified, filtered or spring water alone, but if you elect to do a coffee or tea enema you will need to add two tablespoons of organic fair trade coffee beans or two tablespoons of tea respectively. The most common solution for saline enemas involves two teaspoons of salt to a quart of lukewarm warm.

Other ingredients to consider adding are pure castile soap, vinegar, baking soda, bath/Epsom salt, or mineral oils. These additives are used for the their soothing and beneficial qualities.

Which one you choose depends on the approach you prefer and your circumstances, as there are slight differences in the way each solution works. For example, if you are constipated or have been taking laxatives then your bowel might be irritated enough and it is best to not add any other ingredients to your enema besides water.

The main difference between coffee enemas and the others is the presence of caffeine. Caffeine is more robust in clearing the gastro-intestinal track, removing bile and toxins and stimulating the liver to create more gluthathione. Gluthathione is said to be the mother of all antioxidants, assisting in

185

intracellular DNA health and eliminating toxins residing inside the cells. However, if you have an allergy to coffee the decision of which enemas to choose just got a little bit easier since you should definitely stay away.

Saline and plain water enemas are the mildest options and they work by trying to break up the stool and liquidate it. Normal saline (0.9% sodium chloride) is an isotonic solution, so it does not pull electrolytes from the body. Using this solution reduces the risk of electrolyte imbalance.

People who need to avoid or minimize straining when having a bowel movement can use mineral oil, liquid petroleum or castor oil enemas. They work by lubricating the rectum and help soften impacted stool so that it can slide through the colon easier.

I mentioned the option of purchasing an enema kit with all the bells and whistles already assembled for you if you don't feel up to individually gathering all of your supplies before. Well, that convenience also extends to mixing your solution with the advent of pre-filled enema bags. The market leader for such bags is a company called Fleet Laboratories. They offer multiple options from saline, to mineral oil to sodium phosphate enemas that you can choose from.

Before diving in to the actual steps of your enema, there is some preliminary work that should be done, such as drinking an adequate amount of water because having an enema can be dehydrating. Also, ideally you will want to do your enema after a bowel movement, so you can retain the solution for longer. For this reason, mornings are best for most people. If you are constipated, do the enema anyway - this will get things moving nicely!

After you have completed the above, it is time to make your solution – that is of course unless you will be using a bag that has been pre-filled for you.

For the saline and mineral oil solution, making the final product is a matter of mixing the ingredients into water. If you are doing a tea or coffee enema, put two tablespoons of organic coffee or tea in a saucepan. Add three cups of filtered water and bring to a boil.

Let simmer for fifteen minutes before removing from heat and let it cool. When it's warm - you can test this by placing a clean finger into the coffee, it will be neither hot or cold - strain the mixture through a nut milk bag into a clean glass jar.

Head to the bathroom with your strained or mixed solution and set up a space and something comfortable for you to lie down on. You should be near a toilet. Grab a pillow and some reading material, as you will be here for a little while and you might want to get comfortable.

Now assemble your enema kit. It must have a tube and nozzle attached to the bucket or bag. Make sure it is at least one meter above ground. Hanging the tube on a towel rail or shower rail is a good idea.

There will an attachment near the nozzle that allows you to stop or start the flow of the solution once you have poured it into the bag or bucket. Ensure this is in the off position beforehand.

Once the liquid is in the bag or bucket hold the tube and nozzle over the sink or shower plug and turn it on, allowing the solution to run through the tube until there are no air bubbles. Stop the flow again once this is done.

Grab some lubricant or coconut oil and apply to the nozzle and anus for ease of insertion. Lie down on your towel on your right hand side with your knees drawn up to your chest. The knee chest position allows the solution to flow smoothly into the colon making it easier to fill the entire colon.

Without using force insert the nozzle till it is about two to four inches inside the rectum. Turn on the flow of coffee slowly until the bag or bucket is emptied. Some coffee enema protocols recommend inserting the colon tube twelve to eighteen inches into the colon. However, trying to work a tube this far into the colon is tricky, unnecessary, and possibly counterproductive.

The further you work a tube into your colon, the greater the chances of injuring the colon wall or creating some sort of negative reaction to the tube's material (silicone should be safe). As long as the lower colon has been cleared via a bowel movement or preliminary plain water enema, the fluid will get to where it needs to be with a tube/nozzle insertion of about four inches (or perhaps a little more depending on your body shape and size). That's all it takes.

Now you can either remain lying on your right side or lie on your back with your feet up above head level or feet resting against a wall above head level. You can even do some yoga moves like a shoulder stand or a half plough type position; this helps get the coffee moving round nicely. Just a heads up, you may also hear some funny squirting noises from your tummy, this is a good sign and an indication of the bile being stimulated for release.

Try to retain the enema for twelve to fifteen minutes. You may feel some strong urges to go to the toilet, especially the first few times you try this but try to hold on for as long as you can because quite often the sensation to go will pass. As you do them more regularly you will be able to retain for longer. Fifteen minutes max is all you need.

It is important to remember that enemas should never hurt beyond some mild cramping. If you never use force to administer or retain your enema the threat of stretching the large intestine is essentially eliminated.

When you are ready to release, head to the toilet and let it go. You should feel a lot lighter in body and mind, and the scale should reflect that lightness in a very tangible way. To keep your enema kit in tip-top shape, clean with a mild detergent and ensure everything is dry before packing away.

Remember, enemas are not an end-all weight loss treatment, but rather a tool to be used as part of a comprehensive plan. In general, if you follow the instruction above and use enemas in moderation, you have an exceptional tool to help you reach your weight goals that much faster and improve your physique that has minimal risk.

Colonics

The topic of enemas provide for an easy segue to its sister treatment - the colonic. A colonic, also called colonic hydrotherapy or colon irrigation, is the infusion of water into the rectum by a colon therapist to cleanse and flush out the colon. Sound familiar? It should.

Colonics are a lot like enemas not only in function but also in its popularity. One of the earliest proponents of colonics credited with the widespread popularity of the practice is someone you may have heard of before – Harvey Kellogg, M.D., and founder of the Kellogg cereal company. And in recent years celebrities, spas and wellness facilities have brought these cleanses back to the forefront.

Given colonics and enemas serve the same purpose, they should be treated as substitutes rather than complements. In other words, you should figure out which one you prefer and choose to do one or the other at a time. Do not use the fact that they have different names and slight variations in the process as an excuse to go overboard.

The guideline for how often you should use either treatment applies as though they were one and the same. In other words, since you wouldn't do an enema or colonic daily, you should rotate each treatment on consecutive days and you definitely should not do one after the other back to back. Doing so would result in overtaxing the body and put you at risk for all the negative side effects mentioned before.

Since we have already covered in great detail how cleansing the colon leads to weight loss via enemas and the same remains true for colonics, there is no need to rehash those points. Instead we will address the question that the majority of you will be asking yourself - what are the key differences between a colonic and an enema and which treatment is best for you?

To illustrate the difference in the procedure itself, it might be helpful to start by simply giving you a step-by-step overview of the process for a colonic while pointing out the differences as compared to enemas as we go along. Let's start from the very beginning with the preparation stage.

A day or two before your appointment you should eat light, e.g. non-cream soups or stews with lots of vegetable, fruit, chicken, fish, etc. Staying away from red meat and seafood is advisable as well as avoiding gas producing vegetables and carbonation (e.g., pop, beer, sparkling water). Alcohol and excessive sugars should be cut out completely.

Eating a meal, two to four hours before your colonic is ideal, but no food or beverage should be consumed in the two hours before your appointment. Staying hydrated by drinking a few liters of water throughout the day and the day before your session is also very important in this stage, as it is with enemas.

All colonics must be administered by a trained colon hydrotherapist and requires professional equipment. As you already know, enemas have no such stipulation, are readily available online and in drug stores, and can be administered by yourself as well as a professional.

During the colonic session, you will lay down while warm, filtered water is slowly released into the colon through a tube inserted in the rectum. The tube is about the circumference of your pinky finger and should not hurt much. Here we identify another difference between colonics and enemas with the former involving multiple infusions of water into the colon, and the latter requiring a single infusion of water into the colon.

The water causes the muscles of the colon to contract, called peristalsis. Peristalsis pushes feces out through the hose and unlike the enema, where one has to hold the solution before letting go, the colonic allows for your fecal matter to involuntarily flow out of you without having to lift a finger.

This is yet another one of the key differentiators between the two procedures. As illustrated by the water sitting in the lower part of the colon for a period of time, and then being released, enemas cleanse the lower part of the colon, the sigmoid and part of the descending colon while colonics do a more thorough job by cleansing the entire length of the colon.

As the water flushes out the colon, the fecal matter is disposed in a closed waste system. Such a system ensures the client and the colon therapist do not smell the feces. In comparison enemas would be considered an open waste system.

The therapist will usually look at the feces through the clear hose, and may comment on the color. Depending on the office or the way you are positioned, you may or may not be able to observe along with the therapist.

Another point worth mentioning is that the colon therapist may apply oil, heat or light massage to your abdominal area to help facilitate the bowel movement. This works very well and in fact will be covered in greater detail later on as a weight loss strategy in its own right. The client typically feels some discomfort in the abdomen during the therapy, but generally the experience is pain free.

After the session, which typically lasts forty-five minutes to one hour, the therapist leaves the room, and you may sit on a toilet to pass any residual water and stools.

Once everything is said and done, you are supplied with probiotics to repopulate the good bacteria lost along with the bad bacteria during the colonic. Since there is no pain or recovery time, you should be fine to carry on with the remainder of your day (returning to work, running errands, etc.). You will feel energetic, light and in a very positive mood just as you would with an enema.

For the remainder of the day, you should eat light – fresh vegetable juice, steamed vegetables, non-cream-based soup, light fish are all good options. Additionally, eating food that naturally contain probiotics, like sauerkraut or bone broth soup, is a great idea. Again, stay away from alcohol as it will go directly to your head and is too strong fro your freshly cleaned system.

As you can see, while a lot of the two treatments are similar there are a few variables one might consider that could sway the decision towards one procedure over another.

Colonic Massage

Speaking of colonics, if you are not keen on the invasive nature of the procedure but would like to experience the benefits of lost weight via emptying the colon, you could try doing a colonic massage instead.

As previously mentioned, a colonic massage is commonly given by technicians during the colonic to get your bowels moving along and it really works! Luckily, you don't need to be a professional to master the technique yourself with great results. It's easy and quick - the complete massage should only take about ten minutes. For the best relief, practice it a few times a day.

For this massage, you will be following the path that fecal matter travels in your colon to assist it on its way out. You can choose to either lie down or stand up and use lotion, oil or nothing at all (dry massage). You can even perform your massage in the shower as soap and water will allow for a nice massage motion to occur. Without further ado, here's how to do it.

The first thing to be aware of and master is your touch. The goal is to loosen the fecal matter up and get it out of there so you want to make sure to apply pressure slowly and easily, progressively applying more force if necessary. Be careful not to let the pressure get too hard though, as this can compact the fecal matter further and possibly result in more stagnant matter.

With that in mind, starting near your appendix at the lowest right side of your tummy or around your hipbone, begin applying pressure (a closed fisted massage with the knuckles is best) in small circular movements looking for tension spots. This particular spot is near the ileocecal valve, a sphincter between the small and large intestine in which food must pass through to be further processed in the large intestine. Proper function of this muscle is critical.

An unhealthy ileocecal valve can malfunction and stay closed, hindering in the elimination of waste and providing for a very toxic environment. An unhealthy ileocecal valve can also malfunction by staying open, which causes a backwash of fecal matter from the large intestine into the small intestine. Either dysfunction of the ileocecal valve is toxic, so a healthy ileocecal valve is imperative.

Next, working clock wise, move upwards towards your rib cage continuing to use small circular motions. Using the same directional pattern work your way across the abdomen.

Continue with the small circles and work towards the spot just below your left rib. Continue downwards until you have reached your groin area.

There is no reason to run through the massage. Take your time and massage each area for about one to two minutes before moving on to the next area. If you are in a rush because of time constraints, wait until you will be able to do a thorough job or budget the practice into your schedule just as you would make time to do other things that are important to you.

Note you can employ this massage technique alongside any of the other treatments and strategies mentioned throughout the book. There are really no drawbacks to doing it, so you have everything to gain, including the toning of your abs.

Of course, when practicing this massage if you feel any areas to be particularly painful or if a deep pain persists, consult a doctor as it could signify an underlining issue with your system that should be investigated by a professional.

Diuretics

As discussed in the section on caffeine, a diuretic is any substance that promotes the production of urine. Sometimes called a water pill, diuretics encourage urination by forcing your kidneys to dump lots of water or by preventing sodium absorption, so the excess sodium in the body is then removed in the urine. As a result the appearance of bloating and water weight is reduced.

Diuretics are often used medicinally to address edema (excessive storage of fluid) caused by heart, kidney or liver disease. While some people may take no issue with medical help, others would rather lose less water weight and keep things one hundred percent natural.

There's nothing wrong with having a preference, and as a person who shies away from pills and drugs myself, if you would rather not take any medication some foods/drinks that are natural diuretics include caffeinated drinks such as coffee and tea, apple cider vinegar, cranberries, garlic, artichokes, celery and celery seed (do not take if you are pregnant). The fact that these foods have high water content is probably the main reason they work as a diuretic, but some of them also boost kidney performance as well.

Herbal diuretics like parsley, rosemary, stinging nettle leaf, cleavers, watercress, horsetail, and fennel can be eaten in leaf/herb form or the fresh leaves can be steeped in hot water and consumed as tea.

Typically taken in a more processed form, but perhaps still less unsettling than pharmaceutical diuretics, are nutritional supplements and oils such as evening primrose oil, juniper oil, buchu extract, horse chestnut (should never be eaten raw) and ginkgo (the seed should not be eaten). White kidney bean extract, which eliminates sixty six percent of starch absorption when taken for a short period of time is also a popular staple amongst body builders and dieters as a weight loss aid.

These should all stimulate urine output and many of the flavonoids isolated from the herbs and citrus can also increase the effect, but by far, the two most powerful and widely studied herbal diuretics are goldenrod and dandelion leaf.

According to an animal study published in Planta Medica in 1974, dandelion leaves directly increases urine production on the level of conventional prescription diuretics; As for goldenrod, several studies published by the European Scientific Cooperative on Phytotherapy in 1996 confirmed that it stimulates the kidneys to promote diuretic actions.

That being said, there's no denying that if you want to turbo boost your water weight loss, medical diuretics can help you get the job done without a shadow of a doubt. There are three kinds to choose from, each interacting with the kidneys in a different way: Thiazides, loop diuretics, and potassium-sparing diuretics.

Thiazides or osmotic diuretics are drugs that essentially instruct the kidneys to release everything that comes in nondiscriminately, regardless of proper electrolyte balance. These drugs are not very common amongst dieters.

Potassium sparing diuretics are milder in that they reduce the re-absorption of sodium and water through the kidneys and flush them out, but spare potassium in the process (as the name suggests).

Often prescribed in combination with thiazides or loop diuretics since they are pretty weak on their own, and to help keep the right amount of potassium in your blood while helping other diuretics remove fluid from the body, these diuretics are slower acting with little side effects when routine low doses are used. However, taken alone and/or if abused, they can cause irregular heartbeats due to the excess potassium in the body causing the electrolytes to be unbalanced.

Potassium-sparing diuretics should not be taken by anyone with high levels of potassium in their blood, severe kidney problems or Addison's disease. They should also not be taken potassium supplements or some salt substitutes that are high in potassium.

Lastly, loop diuretics are probably the most powerful and therefore most commonly used type of diuretic because they work so fast (although for a short duration). It should come as no surprise then that the biggest and meanest diuretic of them all can be extremely dangerous. These diuretics are also non-discriminatory and remove all fluids coming through the kidneys, but unlike potassium sparing diuretics they flush potassium, sodium, and calcium from the body with whatever fluid enters.

For weight loss purposes, it is probably safest to start off with natural diuretics (dandelion and goldenrod) since the results are comparable to pharmaceutical drugs and are largely safe. The next most conservative approach is potassium-sparing diuretics taken by itself, followed by mixing potassium sparing diuretics with loop diuretics – taken in small dosages (follow the dosage on your prescription label).

For the most aggressive approach, the use of loop diuretics can be used but must be done with extreme caution, as it doesn't take much for them to cause extremely detrimental health effects - especially paired with other water reduction techniques mentioned in this book.

Either path you decide to take, use of diuretic supplements should be stopped about twenty-four hours before weigh in or when ever you plan on debuting your new physique. This is around the same time you would stop consuming water, sauna treatments, and buckle down with last minute prep for the push to the end (especially if you still have a little weight left to lose before your goal).

The dangers of using diuretics are dehydration, pairing it with other drugs or under conditions that are not recommended by the company, and too much or too little potassium levels in the body depending on the diuretic you take as discussed. Additionally, abusing diuretics can, in the long term, cause renal damage (damage to the kidneys) and of course long-term tolerance can occur in people who take diuretics over a long period of time. Therefore, as with all the other short-term quick weight loss tools featured in this book, use responsibly.

Fasting

Fasting is an age-old practice often done for religious reasons, but fasting for weight loss has captured the public's attention for good reason. Out of all the techniques mentioned this is by far one of the most obvious and foolproof ways to lose an immense amount of weight fast.

The reason is because our bodies need energy to operate and in the absence of food or drinks supplying calories for the body to burn, it will draw on its energy stores (fat/muscle) to get the job done. In the short term, water comes into play as your carb stores are depleted – which explains why weight loss occurs more drastically in the early days of a fast then declines as the fast progresses.

The benefits of fasting don't stop at creating a large caloric deficit for weight loss though. Place under the pro column the fact that it also offers a unique vantage point from which to view your life. Thusly, it's effects aren't just physical, but allow greater understanding and clarity on mental and emotional issues and will make the subsequence changes you need to make in your behavior and lifestyle easier as new decisions flow from you naturally.

In this respect, fasting is almost like pressing the reset button on your tastes, body and mind. It does so by cleansing your palette of chemicals and impurities, giving you a keener ability to fully taste foods and more fully enjoy the true flavors of simple foods. In fact, many people often report the over processed and bad foods they were once addicted to no longer hold the same appeal after a fast. Your body gets reset as well because your stomach actually shrinks so you need less to be full and your digestive system isn't as stressed.

If the above benefits sound attractive to you and you want to give fasting a try, there are a myriad of fasting plans to choose from. This is because fasting quite simply means abstaining from all or some kinds of food or drinks and does not impose strict limitations on the time period that you are required to do so.

To help you sort out all the options and get started, you'll find the five most popular fasting methods and the basics of how they work below. Keep in mind, fasting isn't for everyone, and those with health conditions of any kind should check with their doctor before changing up their usual routine. It's also important to note that personal goals and lifestyle are key factors to consider when choosing a fasting method.

Types of Fasts

Let's begin with probably the most straightforward regimen and what people think of when they hear the word fasting, with what is known as an absolute fast. This is normally defined as no food or liquid for a specific period – usually a single day (twenty-four hours) or several days. It is by far the most difficult to adhere to because there is no reprieve, as you will soon see exists in other protocols, meaning you must exercise a lot more self-control and discipline.

Another type of fasting method – my personal favorite - which has become immensely popular in recent years thanks to Martain Berkhan of the website *Lean Gains*, is intermittent fasting. This is where you have a specific eating window to consume an undefined amount of calories and a specific fasting window where no food or drink is consumed except water.

The recommended fasting period is fourteen hours each day for women and sixteen hours each day for men; Yes, this way of eating is done daily. Most practitioners will find it easiest to fast through the night and into the morning thereby delaying breakfast (which literally stands for breaking a fast and does not correlate to a specific time of day) and eat their first meal around noon.

Simple math deduction dictates that women can feed for the remaining ten hours in the day and men for eight. That being said, some people opt to do longer or shorter feasting/fasting hours without much impact on their success due to their schedules, goals or how they feel. It is not uncommon to do an acclimation period before embarking on the full on system so if you feel the need to break a little earlier than recommended or keep going, you are welcome to do so.

When it's time to eat, the lean gains style of fasting recommends calorie consumption be higher on workout days and lower on rest days but there is no specific calorie intake promoted by the program. However, if you are hoping to cut weight it makes sense to have a calorie deficit at the end of the day.

Understand that just because your feeding hours have been reduced doesn't mean that your diet has now become a free-for-all. You will still gain weight if you consistently eat over

205

your maintenance calories, no matter how narrow your feeding window is. Intermittent fasting is effective, but it isn't magic.

What many people love about this protocol is they don't have to endure a full day of fasting and the time spent not eating feels even easier to tolerate since oftentimes most of the fasting is done overnight. Also, the flexible parameters allow followers to really eat whenever they want within their feasting window. Some also credit the daily routine as being easier to stick to since their hunger cues adapt to the new pattern of eating.

Other noteworthy advantages to this style of fasting is that the time constraints simplifies one's day (preparing less meals), and help thwart overconsumption provided you are eating unprocessed whole foods, as trying to pack all the food in your fridge into a short eating window results in feeling sick and uncomfortable.

Yet another fasting plan that has gained momentum in recent years, made popular by the book, *'Eat, Stop, Eat'* by Brad Pilon, is also termed intermittent fasting. However, the protocol differs in that you must avoid eating for twenty-four hours once or twice a week. The fast can begin in the morning, at lunch or at dinner, as long as you don't eat for a full twenty-four hours. When you do eat and break the fast it is with a normal sized meal.

The next type of fasting is often used in lab studies and by people who have trouble going to bed hungry, and is called alternate day fasting. James Johnson, M.D., is credited as founding alternate day fasting, and as the name suggests, following this method requires eating very little one day and eating like normal the next, before repeating the sequence.

On low-calorie days, that means around one fifth of your normal calorie intake, with your normal intake being maintenance or a small deficit. To give you an idea of a typical eating schedule on this plan, you might have you last meal at, say, 9pm Monday, won't eat the following day and resume eating the day after that at, say, 9am Wednesday.

This works out to around a thirty-six hour fast three or four times a week, depending on whether you start your week on a low or a normal day. Of course, there's a little bit of wiggle room – for example, you could break the fast a little earlier on Wednesday, at, say, 6am for a mere thirty-three hour fast. Either way, fat loss city here you come!

While this method is pretty easy to follow since you do get to consume some food on your fast day and mentally you might be able to withstand the fast better knowing you can eat a much more robust meal, it can be easy to bing on your normal day. The best way to avoid falling off the wagon is to plan meals ahead of time, and make those low calorie day meals as nutrient dense as possible.

Rounding out the top five fasting methods is a style known as the fast diet, promoted in the book, *"The 5:2 fast diet"*. It is somewhat of a combination of alternate day fasting and '*Eat, Stop, Eat*' because it promotes five days of normal eating, but instead of two days of twenty-four hour fasts, the fast diet recommends two days of reduced calorie intake (500 calories for women and 600 calories for men).

Any two days out of the week can be designated as the days in which you lower your calories, meaning you can do two days in a row or space the days out accordingly. The benefits of fast fives lies in the reprieve you get by being able to eat something on your fasting days, without having to fast as frequently as alternate day fasting suggests.

Whew! Believe it or not I could go on and list a few more methods but these five techniques are by far the most lauded. Plus, if you always thought weeks of absolute fasting was the only game in town, these new options now available for you to choose from might already feel overwhelming and confusing.

I know it's a lot to digest but in reality each method is just a slight variation on an initially solid concept, with each style striving to make fasting a bit more accessible to the masses. I speak from experience when I emphatically say that one-day and half day fasts have succeeded in bringing about many internal and external changes for many people, and I guarantee one of these fasting plans will help you get a few steps closer to where you want to be.

That being said, it is simply human nature to want to be told precisely which fasting technique to do, or label things into a tidy hierarchy so that the obvious best choice emerges. I'm sorry to disappoint, but unfortunately the answer is not as cut and dry as you would think or hope.

For example, you might assume that doing two full twenty-four hour fasts would result in more weight loss than daily fourteen to sixteen hour fasts but you would not necessarily be right. Fasting two times per week for twenty-four hours cuts your calorie intake by about thirty percent. However, as long as you cut the same amount of calories on average through any other variation of fasting you will lose about the same amount of weight.

What should be mainly considering is whether or not it would be harder to personally stick to lower calories daily to get to that thirty percent deficit overall, or if eating higher amounts on most days while sacrificing food all day a couple of times a week makes you feel a lot more sane.

The reason I say this is because going a full twenty-four hours without food is a much tougher slog for some people than others. Going lower-carb and higher fat seems to make longer fasts easier, so if you are already used to eating in such a manner, two full days of fasting might just work out better for you. On the other hand if you haven't adapted or yet conditioned to eating whole unprocessed foods on your feasting days or during your eating window, longer fasts will probably be nothing short of a nightmare.

So, the moral of the story is your individual goals, willpower and history (if all day fasting has triggered disordered eating after you end the fast in the past then you might want to try the other methods) really comes into play in your decision-making.

With that said, while all types of fasting will surely lead to weight loss (what you eat after fasting is where the problem arises), and similar calorie deficits over a specific period of time will result in about the same amount of weight loss, how much you lose and how quickly you lose it in shorter time spans can vary depending on which regimen you ultimately choose.

To illustrate my point, if you only have a few days before you need to look your absolute best or weigh in, employing the absolute fasting method for a multitude of days or at least a full day will yield higher weight loss than other options that allow for some consumption. The explanation is fairly straightforward, zero calories a day versus five hundred calories a day will equate to a bigger deficit.

To give you more concrete numbers and a frame of reference, during an absolute fast, women generally lose about fourteen ounces per day and men, on average, lose seventeen and a half ounces per day. This is an average, meaning some days you may lose nothing.

With a fasting plan that includes a small amount of calories, the average amount of weight loss predictably falls. At around two hundred calories per day the figures lower by about 1 ¾ ounces per day, and with a fasting plan including anywhere from 650 to 1300 calories, the numbers drop even more.

There's just no escaping the formula for calories in versus calories out, and if we're talking about time frames being equal – accounting for the fact that you should not do an absolute fast for more than three days (any more is considered the point of diminishing returns because your metabolism slows and muscles get catabolized), it's hard to catch up to such a huge deficit with any of the other fasting methods.

Please do not think the previous statements mean programs like intermittent fasting, alternate day fasting, and 5:2 fasting - where you consume a higher number of calories, should not be an option when you have very little time to prepare. As I said before, there's no one right or wrong plan and there are more variable you have to factor in.

A few of those variables include the commonality for people to experience very low energy levels, which lead to dramatically decreased activity levels, and increased or nearly insatiable appetites upon returning to eating (which may be in the middle of when they were supposed to be fasting). The usual suspects can be attributed to long-term absolute fasts or full day fasts multiple times a week.

Therefore, the side effects of any fasting program and your mental/physical health should be evaluated and held paramount before choosing to just hold out for the longest time or rack up the biggest amount of fasting hours. Specifically, some points to consider include your personality, lifestyle, weight loss goals, the other weight loss strategies you plan on implementing, your current eating habits, etc. In other words, don't make a rash decision based on emotion alone.

The fact of the matter is, if you can't adhere to a more aggressive program you would be better off with a conservative one that you can stick to. Some results trump no results, wouldn't you say?

HOW TO MASTER FASTING

As alluded to in the things you need to consider before choosing the right fasting plan, it is quite one thing to want to fast to lose weight and another to successfully do so. This is especially true since we need to eat to live and we live in a culture where food is abundant and we have been conditioned to eat regularly. Going without food for an extended period of time, even if it's only fourteen hours (the recommended bare minimum in all of the five protocols mentioned), can seem darn near impossible.

For those who have bought into the dogma of grazing all throughout the day as the healthiest and best way to eat – e.g. three larger meals and two snacks, or five to seven small meals in what works out to a meal every two hours or so for most, adjusting to fasting will probably prove the most difficult. It's no surprise either, as their bodies, hunger cues and digestive systems have become used to their eating pattern and will initially revolt against not being fed according to its expectations.

Despite all of this, we ultimately have the power to control our actions and change our habits over time so don't be discouraged if you currently fit the description of an all day grazer. Remember, many people with very different eating habits – one of which closely resembles your current one, have faced and worked out the kinks of fasting before you (again, this is a method as old as the bible).

Even more encouraging news is that such accounts have been graciously recorded and shared so that luckily, you don't have to pioneer the path and can instead be guided along it with the equivalent of a foolproof tourist's map. You can learn from other's mistakes and successes to make the transition to fasting as seamless and pain free as possible.

I will share five of the most common challenges expressed by experienced fasters as well as their tips and tricks for beating them with you now; the idea being if you know how the enemy will attack you can take the necessary action to defend yourself and come out the victor or at least avoid turning into the incredible hulk out of hunger.

As promised, the five most common difficulties that accompany fasting are: feelings of hunger (shocker, right?), fatigue and brain fog, headache, sensitivity to cold, and trouble falling asleep.

I know, enduring hunger and not being able to at least escape it with the aid of sleep is definitely not what you want to hear. To prevent you from abandoning the idea of fasting altogether, it's worth mentioning that you are not guaranteed to encounter every single item on the list and that most of the symptoms, if they appear, are usually transient.

214

Everybody reacts to fasting slightly differently, and the length of the fast will surely affect the degree to which you experience problems along the way. Besides, there's no reason to fret because I will now reveal the best-proven defenses against these obstacles.

Feelings of Hunger

Without a doubt, the biggest complaint all fasters will encounter at first is feelings of hunger. A lot of times the feeling is more mental than physical and is triggered by what you surround yourself with.

To speak to the mental aspect first, it would do you well to remove all reminders and possible temptations of food. Some actions you can take include cleaning out your fridge and cupboards and letting the people in your life who like to surprise you with food know you are fasting so you won't have to test your will by declining their latest treat. If this happens often in your place of work stay out of the kitchen or if the food is brought into a common area, avoid eye contact – seriously, we tend to get hungry with our eyes.

More tips to beat your brain hunger is to avoid cooking for others if possible - this might be hard if you have a family but perhaps trying cooking them food that you hate/dislike that

215

they don't mind eating). Stop hanging around in coffee shops and other places with your favorite eats, and definitely do not agree to dine out with friends (if you think you can nurse a water while your friend eats appetizers, dinner and dessert without caving you are lying to yourself). As an added precaution, do not carry more cash than you need to get around - ditch the credit card or leave it in the car to ensure you won't buy food on a whim.

That should take care of the mentally brought on feelings of hunger, but what about when true physical hunger rears its magnificent head and manifests in belly growling and churning? The first defense is to keep your mouth occupied by sucking on some cold ice, or drinking tea or ice-cold water.

The second defense is to keep your brain occupied – ideally by engaging in an activity that you really enjoy doing. Have you ever noticed that children are never hungry when they are outside playing with their friends, but when they are stuck in the house all you hear is "I'm hungry," or "I'm thirsty"? That's the power of keeping busy in action.

The reason this works is distractions remove the boredom one feels from the inability to entertain one's self with food – even for those who are not addicted to food. Honestly, the desire to eat is not just about curbing hunger. It's about being social, releasing endorphins which makes one happy and escaping the daily routines / chores we are faced with. All of these things are lost on a fast, so knowing in advance how you will fill the role food used to play whenever boredom rears its ugly head is essential.

Finally, you can proactively fight hunger a lot more effectively by preparing for your fast in advance as much as possible. I said it before and I'll repeat it again - those who go into fasting with a diet background higher in unprocessed whole foods as well as fat and protein, and lower in carbohydrates and junk food tend to fare much better.

This is especially important if you are doing intermittent fasting because the things you eat during your eating window, such as (sugars, grains, etc.) can really stoke the fire of your appetite. Poor nutrition will cause cravings and that spells disaster when fasting.

If the hunger and cravings gets too intense then break your fast and eat something. Don't feel bad and just try to fast a little longer the next time until you hit the desired hour range of your specific protocol or even test out a different plan altogether.

Fatigue and Brain Fog

Physical fatigue as a result of fasting means feeling tired because your energy reserves are temporarily depleted. You might even find the idea of eating appealing not so much because of cravings but to get an energy boost.

Brain fog, which is not a medically recognized term, is a commonly used phrase that succinctly sums up feelings of confusion, forgetfulness, and lack of focus and mental clarity. Basically, you feel like you just can't think, which can be very frustrating and puts a stop to trying to keep yourself busy as a way of beating the problem because you lack the energy to do so.

On the bright side, both symptoms subside when you have been following fasting for a while; during a twenty-four hour fast, they start to subside after an hour or so. Unfortunately, when you are actually faced with either feeling and they are affecting your ability to do your job or much of anything else, such statements probably offer very little in terms of comfort.

So what can you actually do to lift the fog? As previously mentioned, one of the effects of fasting is not being able to sleep. Well guess what? Lack of restorative sleep leads to fog and fatigue. The fact that fasting causes problems sleeping, which causes brain fog, might seem like an insurmountable loop that can only be broken by stopping the fast, but it's not.

I'll get to how to solve problems falling asleep while fasting in its own section, but for now, suffice to say that sleep as well as preventing disruptions in the deep sleep patterns that prevent the limbic system from recharging will do a lot to combat this issue.

Additionally, although it might seem like the answer to almost everything, making sure your diet is in check while not fasting and that you are drinking plenty of water, water and more water really does help. A number of nutrient-dense foods with specific anti-inflammatory qualities, such as green vegetables, sprouted grains and legumes, and healthy fats, are shown to support brain health and cognitive function.

On the other hand, junk foods high in sugars and trans fats fuel inflammation and impair cognitive function. Worse, insulin dysfunction, usually related to chronically elevated blood sugar from an unhealthy diet, is a major risk factor in dementia and cognitive decline. So, reigning in your diet will do well to quell inflammation, thereby helping to lift brain fog.

Besides restorative and uninterrupted sleep, diet and hydration, another one of the underlying issues of brain fog is an inability to get oxygen and nutrients to the brain. Many times this comes down to a circulation issue, which can be related to a sedentary lifestyle, lack of exercise, and other factors.

The remedy? Regular exercise. It increases neural connections throughout your body, balances hormones, and supports numerous other aspects of health. Studies now show that one of the most important things you can do for your brain is to get up and move around - go for regular walks, take bike rides, get out in nature. If you find yourself stuck in a fog, get out and exercise, and notice the clarity you feel afterwards.

Headache

The next top issue faced by a lot of people, especially with their first one or two fasts, is headaches or even migraine. There are two reasons this happens. The first reason – dehydration as a result of not drinking enough fluids, should come as no surprise by now. Food contains a lot of water so by not eating we are not taking in as much water. You need to drink far more than you think in order to compensate for the lack of water you are having in food.

In case you didn't realize a pattern emerging in the solutions being given, water (and tea) should become your BFF when undertaking fasting if you want to cut down on the negative side effects many people experience.

The second cause of headaches while fasting is low blood sugar. Although the body has a great system for swapping between glucose as a fuel to glycogen stores and eventually to fat stores, when we are overweight the body is reluctant to swap to fat burning. This is at least partly due to high insulin levels, which act to prevent the fat stores being mobilized.

Because the body is slow to swap to fat burning, it fails to compensate for the lack of glucose in the blood (by producing ketone bodies through fat burning). The resulting low blood sugar combined with no ketone bodies leaves the brain short of fuel and triggers a headache.

Over time, the body will eventually become fat adapted and the headaches will diminish with each resulting fast, eventually disappearing altogether. This means your options are to keep eating high carb and risk attendant obesity problems, wait out the headaches, or try to enter a state of ketosis. If you choose to go with the latter, the best way to do so is to eat a low carb diet at least on the day before a fast and do some exercise while fasting.

Cold Sensitivity

This one is probably the easiest to solve of all the fasting complaints. An increased sensitivity to cold is a common problem with those who practice chronic calorie restriction, but the "less energy, less body heat" rule applies to fasting as well.

It's natural for the body to respond to fasting by down regulating activity and metabolism to converse energy.

However, in the case of short-term fasts, the effect is only temporary. During the first twelve hours of the fast, nothing really significant happens, but from there on, the sensitivity to cold begins to make its appearance. The most pronounced effect is seen towards the end of the twenty-four hour fast.

Some suggestions for nipping the cold in the bud while fasting include wearing another layer of clothes or warmer clothes in general (wool socks, gloves, heck – maybe even think about bringing the turtleneck back in style!), moving more (exercise), drinking hot tea, turning up the thermostat, taking a warm bath and focusing on soups when you are in the eating phase.

For the brave and fearless, contrast hydrotherapy – or the application of heat followed by an application of cold- is also an effective option. You can perform contrast hydrotherapy with a bath or in the shower. All it takes is exposing yourself to heat for three or so minutes, and then switching to cold for one minute. If the thought of standing under ice-cold water scares the daylight out of you, footbaths or heating and cooling pads applied to the chest/neck area can be employed instead.

Lastly, a great hack for warming up simply requires breathing deeply and slowly for five minutes and can be done anywhere or anytime.

Trouble Sleeping

As promised, it's time to focus our attention to the final common fasting related difficulty among those who do longer fasts or have just started to do shorter fasts - trouble falling asleep. Once rectified this will also help those of you suffering from fatigue and brain fog.

One reason many people have trouble falling asleep while fasting has to do with the adjustment the body needs to make once you start going to bed without a dinner or an evening snack. Again, this is not the case for everyone, and some people are able to fall sleep by telling themselves it will take their mind off the hunger!

However, if you can relate to hunger pangs keeping you up at night, using the techniques outlined in dealing with hunger while fasting (keeping your mind and/or body busy with a book, podcast, hot bath, or low intensity workout like yoga, Pilates, or going for a quick walk a short while before bed, drinking water or sucking on ice, etc.) will help.

After an induction period and your body has gotten used to its new eating pattern, going to bed without food should no loner prove to be no problem. You may even find that you sleep better than you did before and need less sleep overall.

Another way to attack this problem is to change your feasting time so that you are eating most of your calories in the evening and fasting in the daytime. If you make the switch be sure that your evening meal is full and satiating, as this will make you sleepy. If this is not an option, you could turn to outside help by buying melatonin, a natural sleep aid available without a prescription, or magnesium tablets. Both are available in most drugstores and pharmacies.

Another scenario you might experience is it being 2:00am and instead of your empty tummy keeping you up, your brain, which might be going a mile a minute, and your boundless levels of energy is the culprit for not being able to get adequate shuteye.

It makes sense when you think about it because with fasting comes an increase in energy as our brains start running on ketones. Ketones are said to be more efficient than glucose. When our insulin resistant brains and bodies start relying on ketones for energy rather than glucose, the result is more energy to our brains, more efficient metabolism and clearer thinking.

This explains why it has been said that Einstein used to fast to gain greater mental clarity.

The moral of the story is all of these functions in your body means you don't actually need as much sleep as you think. So while you can try avoiding drinking caffeine well before bedtime, and/or drinking relaxing teas (such as rooibos) instead, another alternative would be to maximize your increased energy and mental clarity by finding something more productive to do instead of sleeping.

One final word of advice that will take care of a lot of these issues is to seriously avoid going into a fast unprepared – if you've binged on sugar, alcohol, lack of sleep, etc. the day before, a twenty four hour fast is probably not your best bet. When you adequately prepare yourself, you won't have the urge as much to cheat or give up because psychologically and physiologically you'll be in a much stronger place.

Finally, no matter how long you choose to fast, it can be a relief to just to quit eating or thinking about eating for awhile, rather than stressing and worrying over everything you put in your mouth. Most protocols in this book won't have nearly as much flexibility as fasting (it's either you do it one way or you don't do get the benefits at all), so do take advantage of the fact that if one system doesn't jibe with you, you are free to play around with the others until you find something that does.

Juice Cleanse

Maybe it was the Master Cleanse, a crash diet technique that involves drinking nothing but a mixture of water, cayenne pepper, lemon juice and organic maple syrup for ten days to experience rapid weight loss, that started the juice cleanse trend so popular throughout America. After all, celebrities like Beyoncé specifically credited the concoction for helping slim down to her lowest weight thus far for a Hollywood role.

Nowadays, the juice cleanse market in general has grown by leaps and bounds thanks to blessings of approval by high-profile people like Nicole Richie, Salma Hayek, Gwyneth Paltrow, and Dr. Oz, along with a whole host of influential beauty, health and fitness gurus and bloggers.

Chances are you even know an enthusiastic juicing friend or two because everyone has seemingly jumped on the train for the simple reason that they work extremely well for dropping weight fast, resetting eating habits, getting cravings under control and kick starting a healthy lifestyle.

Whatever the cause of the prolific spread of its existence throughout the population thankfully, juice cleanses have evolved from the days where the master cleanse was the ubiquitous choice to include more variety, in terms and ingredients and flexibility. Juice cleanses of today, also known as juice fasting, now ensure people are able to get all of the essential nutrients and vitamins the body needs as well as actually enjoy the taste of the juice in the process.

I can recall watching a news program profile a revolutionary juicing and bottling company delivering and shipping its line of cold pressed juices in coolers to health conscious people in the New York area for a pretty penny (around $60 to $75 a day, not including shipping). Fresh juice is hardly that expensive to actually make and can keep for up to seventy-two hours as long as it's stored in airtight containers and kept refrigerated so the model, which typically offered four to seven juices a day for as little as two days to a full week, did extremely well.

What was once a novel concept is no longer so newsworthy as a slew of companies have entered the market in an attempt to grab a piece of the estimated five-billion dollar and growing industry. The brands that have risen to the top today include BluePrint, Cooler and Ritual Cleanse, but a quick Internet search turned up over 800,000 results for juice cleanse programs, which should tell you that there are no shortage of options.

Meanwhile others have tried to make juice cleanses more accessible to the public in both cost and simpler, more convenient distribution plans. This is why you can now buy pre-bottled one, three and five day juice cleanses from the likes of Suja at big box stores like Costco and Target, or Evolution Fresh at Starbucks and Whole Foods.

Undoubtedly, the neighborhood supermarket, health oriented natural markets or boutique outfits like Organic Avenue and Juice Press, in your area has a line or two for you to choose from as well. It is important to note here that what previously constituted as acceptable juice in cleanses was freshly made and unpasteurized, so the usual bottles of OJ that you would pick up at the corner store wouldn't be allowed on your cleanse. While those markers still stand, new processes have entered the equation.

Most bottled juices, like the aforementioned OJ, are pasteurized, which means they have been heat-treated to kill bacteria. Unfortunately, that process also kills many of the enzymes and phytonutrients in the juice. The juices you mainly see on the shelves of your big chain retailers are not fresh in the sense that the product is older than the natural time it takes to decompose – about twenty five or so days versus the two to four days for cold pressed, but are generally considered fine for a juice cleanse. How so?

This is possible through a process called HPP (High Pressure Processing) that subjects the juice to very high pressure, which inactivates pathogens while helping to retain the flavors of fresh fruits and vegetables. In other words enzymes are not destroyed or killed in the process. If your budget doesn't allow for the more expensive cold pressed juice systems, HPP labeled bottled juices are your next best bet.

That being said, by far the cheapest, beneficial and most controllable type of juice cleanse is one where you use fresh vegetable and fruits – whether you make it on your own or place an order with a barista at your favorite juice bar, and drink that juice right away.

Going this route means you get to choose exactly what mixture of fruits, vegetables, and the rare herbs and spices found from juice manufacturers, like cilantro, parsley, mint, basil, cayenne pepper, ginger and chili powder, make it into your drink. You don't have to worry about undesirable ingredients entering the fray (e.g. added sugar or nuts), or whether everything is all natural when you juice everything yourself - which is why you should definitely make sure to read those labels when it comes to bottled juice purchases.

After all, it would be foolish to assume all cleanses are created equally. While many companies truly promote juicing as a healing and detoxing treatment, others are simply in the game to make money. Everything about their marketing and packaging is to get you to buy even if their product is sub par and will make the fact that it will be all you'll consume for a few days even more dreadful than necessary. There is a drastic difference between the revitalizing mental and wellness boosts from fresh live juice and the lack of such effects from juice stripped of all its goodness after all.

Additionally, since your goal is to lose weight, while you are checking out the ingredients of bottled juices or comprising your recipes, be aware of the calories as well. The New York Times reported that most new cleanses contain about 1,000 to 2,000 calories per day, however some programs might have you ingesting fewer than 500 calories a day while others will bring you over your maintenance amount by including a nut-milk component meant to provide a small amount of fat and protein.

Contrary to popular opinion, fruits and vegetables are not free foods – they contain energy, and you can fit a lot of fruit and vegetable servings in one big glass of juice. Just one glass of fruit juice has the calories of two pieces of whole fruit. Too much a day (some cleanses advocate unlimited juice) and you will see weight gain just as you would over eating any other food.

By and large, most people prefer the yummy sweet aroma and taste of fruits in their juices, more than likely because the majority of fruit is chock full of the irresistible white stuff - sugars. Unfortunately for those looking for an excuse to fuel their sugar addiction in a healthier way via juice treats, you are in for a rude awakening. Because juice doesn't offer the fiber contained in fresh fruits and vegetables, the body absorbs fructose sugar more easily.

If you recall what we know to be true about sugars causing spikes in insulin, blocking fat burning, and enhancing your taste for more sweet stuff - only maybe once you are off your juice fast you might try to scratch the itch with a piece of candy, pack or cookies or plate of cake - you might want to avoid opening Pandora's box in the first place.

This is why I strongly recommend sticking to green juices (kale, spinach, broccoli, cucumber, chard, collard greens, wheatgrass, etc.). If you just can't hack what admittedly isn't the most delicious taste in the world – raw, veggie juice - try to find juices/recipes that include just a small amount of fruit or uses carrots and beets to enhance the taste.

Another area cleansing programs tend to differ is in the recommendation to incorporate eating fresh, whole foods while doing a juice fast. Traditionally juice fasts like the master cleanse did not include solids or whole foods, which is the primary reason people could lose so much weight in so little time. What you must realize is that many cleansing systems on the market today do not tout its weight loss properties as anything but a side effect that might accompany detoxification and healing, therefore the aim to get you consuming ultra low calories does not align with their purpose.

On the other hand, we are using juicing mainly as a push toward last minute quick weight loss. Therefore, while you may certainly choose to substitute one or two meals for a juice to help you reach a lowered calorie and food volume intake, your weight loss will not be as drastic as the five to seven pound losses in a week common to those who undergo juice fasts in its original incarnation.

If you have very little weight to lose, or a longer time to lose the weight that may be fine as long as you realize the result will likely be slower weight loss – which isn't necessarily a bad thing. It really is your call which way you'd like to go. Please note, since you should not be drinking calories or snacking do not simply add juices on top of your regular meals or make them snack replacements.

Clearly, there are a lot of similarities between fasting and juice cleanses. For starters, they both help you accomplish huge weight loss by reducing bloat, encouraging digestion and the purging of waste, and lowering your calories. Weight loss from both protocols is a combination of fat, muscle, and water, but staying active and drinking enough juice and water will help to preserve muscle mass and promote comparatively more fat loss.

Another similarity between the two is probably not the most welcome of news, but nonetheless there's no escaping it; that is you may experience the same challenging symptoms on a juice cleanse as you would with fasting, such as hunger, headaches, cold sensitivity, etc.

However, since it is okay to drink fluids other than water and tea on a juice fast, I would recommend coconut water to restore your electrolytes in addition to drinking copious amounts of water, as most issues are treatable by staying hydrated. You should also refer to the other solutions outlined in the common challenges of fasting section.

Given the similarities you may be confused about which method to use – fasting or a juice cleanse? One really isn't inherently better than the other, but there are some factors that might assist in your decision, where juice fasts and regular fasting go in separate directions is the length of time you can do the protocol without harming yourself.

Since juice cleanses actually involve consuming calories and nutrition, you don't necessarily have to strictly limit the fast to three days or else risk endangering your health and metabolism as you would with absolute fasts. You will find most people doing cleanses for three to five days, but seven, ten, fourteen, twenty-one and even thirty days is possible.

That being the said, it is possible to do a juice cleanse for too long or too often, and undesirable side effects such as nutrition deficiencies or metabolic disruptions are the price you will pay when you cross that threshold.

Therefore, you should always listen to your body when it tells you that it cannot go on while being cognizant to the fact that it is definitely not necessary to go on an extended juice fast to lose a large amount of weight. The initial water weight loss phase tends to be up to seven days, so depending on your unique circumstance anywhere from one to seven days will probably be your sweet spot.

Another departure from regular fasting is that most juice cleanses call for the addition of colonics or enemas during the program. The reasons range from helping to keep the digestive tract open and moving (which is harder to do without roughage and solid foods), to relieving nausea and other detox symptoms, to eliminating the toxins released by the cleanse so that they do not get reabsorbed into the blood.

That about sums up the main contributing factors most individuals use to decide which fasting program is the best fit for their unique circumstances and situation. Whichever one you choose will be effective, so don't stress yourself out too much about which way to go. Just pick one and give it a go. Generally, I would say juicing is probably the best place to start if you've never done absolute fasting before.

Just remember, neither treatment is meant to facilitate healthy long-term weight loss. After your juice cleanse, you can minimize regaining weight by easing into a healthy diet, staying active, and drinking plenty of water – common sense stuff.

Also obvious but needs to be stated - most fruits and vegetables are naturally free of common allergens, such as dairy, soy, wheat and gluten, but if you are allergic, or think you might be, to any fruits or veggies, please do not consume them during your cleanse.

If you take medications, please continue taking them as prescribed, and ask your doctor if you need to make any adjustments. For those of you taking statins to lower cholesterol, please avoid grapefruit. For those taking medication for thyroid conditions, please avoid juicing or eating raw cruciferous vegetables, such as broccoli, cabbage, cauliflower, kale and radish, in large amounts as some of their phytonutrients can interfere with the medication. (It's fine to eat these items cooked.) Also, please check with your pharmacist or doctor about any drug/food interactions you need to be aware of.

Handstands and Inversions

There's no question that improving circulating and accelerating the cleansing of blood and lymph fluids has an effect on water retention. It just so happens that there is a way to accomplish these things in one movement – turning your body upside down.

This practice is better known as inversion therapy and was used as early as 400 B.C., when Hippocrates, the father of medicine, first watched a patient have his knees bound and ankles tied to a ladder to be hoisted upside down for a dose of what's come to be known as spinal traction.

The practice is well-known today as a natural way to a better back and body, but what isn't as widely covered is its ability to flush out waste, promote the healthy exchange of nutrients and help fluids flow more efficiently throughout the body – all properties right up our alley!

For starters, recall what we covered earlier about the lymphatic system being responsible for waste removal, fluid balance and immune system response, and that it also has no pump. Only the alternate contraction and relaxation of muscles moves the fluid upward through capillaries and one-way valves to the upper chest for cleansing and flushing.

Inverting the body so that gravity works with these one-way valves stimulates the entire lymphatic system and helps to push the lactic fluid up to the chest.

The good news is that you don't need to be hanging around all day to see benefits. Remaining inverted for three to five minutes a day is all it takes for the body to improve lymphatic fluid accumulation with results akin to a lymphatic massage or body wrap.

In other words, while you may not see a huge change in your scale weight from doing inversions, you will have a slimmer, more toned overall appearance. You'll fit into clothes better, and if your extremities like your arms and legs are prone to bloating/puffiness (commonly caused by the strain of walking, running and compromised vascular/immune function) there will be a marked difference.

In addition to sorting out the lymphatic system, inversions are great for weight loss by improving digestion and elimination. The change in gravitational pull on the body affects the abdominal organs so that the bowels move freely and the pressing of the stool against the intestinal walls encourages movement. By now it should be apparent how elimination has a direct tie to how much you weight.

An approach a bit more indirect, but still important nonetheless, is how inversions have been known to elevate the mood and relieve depression. It's a no brainer that remaining positive and motivated to lose weight doesn't mesh well with symptoms of depression. So, if you feel yourself getting dejected with your goals turn to inversions.

It increases the circulation and oxygen to the brain, which leads to the release of neurotransmitters, the balancing of hormones, endorphin-releasing movement, and therapeutic postural correction. Believe it or not, but is normal to feel immediately uplifted after a session of inversions, and that's exactly how you should feel throughout your journey if you want to make it across that finish line.

If you're semi-convinced to give inversions a shot but visions of lithe yoga practitioners fill your head along with a pessimistic inner voice about there being no way you'll be able get your body even halfway up in the air, I want you to block all of that noise out and focus squarely on the next few words.

There is more than one way to hang upside down in order to get the benefits of inversion. If you are young and minimally agile gravity boots are one option. They can easily be taken anywhere, any child playground has somewhere to hang, and the rack can be placed indoor and removed. Inversion tables are another option that makes hanging upside down a lot easier. Yes, they are a little bit more expensive, require space, and are not for traveling but they get the job done very easily.

Finally, there's supporting your own body weight with the headstand and shoulder stand, referred to as the king and queen of all yoga asanas, with the headstand being the king and shoulder stand being the queen.

Headstand tends to heat the body and stimulate the nervous system and tones the neck muscles. Shoulder stand tends to cool or neutralize the body and sedate the nervous system while releasing the muscles of the neck and shoulders.

In practice together, the logical sequence is to do headstand first, followed by shoulder stand either immediately after, or later in your practice session. Headstand can leave you feeling very stimulated, so once it is done you really are committed to doing the other. Shoulder stand can be safely practiced on its own as it has the amazing ability to neutralize the nervous system.

These moves might seem very intimidating at first but if you remember that every one started out in the same position you are in now (as a beginner) you'll realize it's only a matter of time before you're the one looking like a pro. I think it's safe to say no one just got up one day without ever doing a headstand/handstand and nailed it without any instruction or a few tumbles.

That's totally okay too and is the reason teachers/classes solely dedicated to helping you hoist your legs above your head exist. You'll learn in baby steps – first with the assistance of the wall or maybe with your knees bent, until you can do the poses unassisted and fully extended. If you can't find an inversion workshop near you, your next best option is to turn to YouTube for video tutorials; this will yield a ton of results. If possible recruit a spotter or a wall and get to work.

As usual, some of you chomping at the bit to take on inversions need to first make sure it's a good fit. People suffering from high blood pressure, detached retina, glaucoma, hernias, cardiovascular disease, cervical spondylitis, slipped discs should not practice shoulder stand. Also, those suffering from neck injuries should seek advice from an experienced yoga teacher before beginning to practice shoulder stand.

A potential problem with inversion therapy is that it may significantly increase blood pressure in your head. For this reason, you should not try inversion therapy if you have heart disease, high blood pressure, eye diseases - such as glaucoma, during menstruation, or if you are pregnant.

Acupuncture & Acupressure

Before you scoff and dismiss the idea of acupuncture or acupressure for weight loss as hogwash, hear me out. As with every other technique I've reviewed thus far, skeptics and naysayers abound (mostly people who have never tried any of the things they claim to be bogus) – that doesn't change the fact that the strategies have helped someone somewhere shed pounds fast and effectively.

The reason I've included acupuncture and acupressure here is because the techniques are safe and sound. Hundreds of thousands of people have seen real results from giving these methods a fair shot because like fasting and colon cleansing, acupuncture for weight loss has been used for centuries - at least 2,500 years, to be exact.

To you, acupuncture/acupressure for weight loss might seem like news as you may only be familiar with stories of the procedures being used to help people stop bed wetting, treat headaches, and/or ease back pain. I also thought the benefits ended at pain alleviation until I personally witnessed acupuncture stop a full-blown asthma attack in a matter of minutes.

If all these ailments can be treated with the same simple underlying principle, which is that balancing and modifying patterns of energy flow through the body that are essential for health to address a wide range of disorders, then why would claims of weight loss seem unreasonable?

Don't get me wrong; if something is good at one thing it will not automatically be good at a bunch of other things too. Clearly that is not true. Also, unless you've personally experienced something for yourself, testimonies like the ones above and all over the Internet serve as nothing but anecdotal accounts in convincing you. The thing is along with controlled trials, anecdotal accounts and understanding the theory behind the way something works are the best markers we have to reasonably determine what to trust and what to ignore.

Given the plethora of trials, anecdotes and the basic theory behind acupuncture and acupressure, it would appear there is something legitimate to this practice that makes it worthy of being mentioned here. Even if the results are simply the placebo effect in action, if a placebo ends up helping me achieve something I wouldn't have otherwise, I say sign me up. Besides, the treatment being relatively cheap, it is much safer than taking untried drugs.

That being said, you may be pleased to learn in my research on how and why the techniques work to help you lose weight I came across several plausible reasons and studies that suggest a placebo has very little to do with the success people experience. In fact, in one study the results seemed to expressly prove that notion.

The study, posted in the online journal "Acupuncture in Medicine", looked at two kinds of ear acupuncture or auricular acupuncture, which was first used in France in 1956 by Dr. Paul Nogier. He noticed that patients' backaches were cured when they received a burn on the ear. Intrigued, he started mapping the ear, pinpointing the spots that correlate to various organs or systems in the body.

Dr. Nogier pictured the ear as a curled up fetus with its head pointing downwards, and began treating his patients by applying pressure to the spot associated with each organ.

For the study ninety-one overweight Koreans were put on the same diet without any additional exercise. Some were given the five-point treatment - five needles placed in five different key points of the ear thought to be linked to the stomach, spleen, endocrine and hunger, others were given the single point treatment - one needle placed in the ear's hunger point – the point linked to appetite, and others still were given a sham treatment - to test the placebo effect.

After four weeks, those in the five-point group showed a 6.1 percent reduction in BMI, while the one point group showed a 5.7 percent reduction, and the sham group showed no reduction at all. On top of that, fifteen participants in the sham treatment group dropped out, suggesting they found it harder to regulate their hunger and cope with the restrictive diet without the aid of acupuncture.

To find out how and why the participants who received treatment were able to drop weight, let's look at some ways that acupuncture is said to help with weight loss.

The idea of acupressure and acupuncture rests on the belief that we have pressure points in the meridians or channels of the body where vital energy (or life force called qi) flows. It is believed that the twelve major meridians connect organs or a system of organs and as previously mentioned, illness occurs when one of the meridians is blocked or unbalanced.

Inserting needles in those specific points act to help balance hormones and stimulate the release of endorphins, the body's natural "feel good" hormones. This can create a more positive, calming, relaxing effect, which counteracts the need for excessive eating brought about by increased stress, frustration or anxiety. In this respect, acupuncture can calm those so afflicted and help them lose weight without resorting to drugs or binge eating.

Aside from balancing hormones and increasing endorphins, acupuncture and acupressure also *reduces* the hormones that lead to overeating, and reduces stress. We already know that the pesky cortisol hormone can affect weight by disrupting digestion, and contributing to depression. Again, it becomes terribly difficult to motivate oneself to eat right and exercise with a cloud of depression looming.

The third way acupuncture is said to lead to weight loss is by aiding digestion through getting the spleen and liver in balance. In Traditional Chinese Medicine, the belief is that

244

excessive weight gains are caused mainly by an imbalance in the body due to a malfunction of the spleen and liver organ systems. Disharmony and imbalance in the spleen can lead to fatigue, slow metabolism, water retention, loose stools, and a feeling of heaviness. On the flip side, disharmony in the liver can lead to cravings and compulsive eating.

Other areas, such as the endocrine system and kidneys are addressed to treat water retention and to stimulate nerve and hormonal rebalance. Additionally, the thyroid glands can also be targeted to effect sugar and hormonal rebalancing. Skilled acupuncture practitioners will zero in on these specific body areas to effect weight loss both physically and psychologically.

All of the above seem to make plausible and compelling arguments for how these treatments can be viewed as a support system for weight loss. There are no absurd claims that putting a needle in your body will poke holes in the fat cells causing them to burst or anything silly like that. We are simply targeting water retention and promoting weight loss in the same ways advocated in other techniques showcased in the book.

For example, restoring hormones and systems in the body that regulate what you ultimately put into your mouth, reducing stress, and addressing metabolic imbalances are all issue we target with diet, massage, inversion therapy, and exercise yet no one would ever dispute these actions can lead to weight loss.

In case you don't have a problem with the idea of giving acupuncture a try, but like me, you are not a fan of long needles, an alternative to acupuncture is acupressure. Both methods stimulate acupoints, but acupuncture uses a hair-thin needle to stimulate the acupoints whereas acupressure uses a firm pressure to massage the acupoints. For the sake of full disclosure, acupuncture will trigger a stronger stimulation to activate the body's innate healing ability than acupressure, but that doesn't make acupressure completely useless.

To prove this point, studies have tested the validity of the beneficial claims associated with acupressure as well. For example, one study used a randomized controlled design to test the effects of auricular acupressure interventions for weight reduction in sixty-eight Taiwanese young adults who ranged in age from eighteen to twenty years old with a BMI greater than 23 kg/m^2. The total intervention duration was four weeks, and all participants were free to withdraw from the study at any time.

The subjects were randomly placed into two groups and all received health education describing an appropriate reduced calorie diet and lifestyle modification. The control group had adhesive tape placed on the ear acupoints, while the experimental group received Semen Vaccariae (small sticks only) for acupressure on the auricular acupoints. All participants met one time per week for ten minutes for a total of four weeks.

After four weeks the BMI of the control group increased significantly by +0.0457 kg/m2 (P = 0.000). Thus, simply applying adhesive tape to ear acupoints could not decrease BMI after four weeks. Meanwhile, the BMI of the treatment group decreased significantly by −0.8022 kg/m2 (P ≤ 0.0001) and were noted to have decreased BMI from week to week.

Another completely needle free option for us scaredy-cats, based in the principles of acupressure, is the practice of finger tapping – otherwise known as the Emotional Freedom Technique (EFT). This practice involves tapping acupoints on the face and body to reduce stress and anxiety levels while equipping the dieter with the mental tools necessary to beat the root cause of cravings and curbing the appetite.

The stimulation of these points supposedly decreases activity in the amygdala – the apart of the brain that controls the production of the stress hormone cortisol – linked to increased appetite, sugar cravings, and abdominal fat levels.

Scientific claims that support finger tapping remain limited, but most tapping and EFT websites refer to a Harvard Medical School study on eighty-nine women that showed those who tapped for fifteen minutes a day lost an average of sixteen pounds in eight weeks, without following a strict diet or exercise plan. Remarkably, they had kept that weight off six months later.

With impressive results like the one I just shared, you should be pleased to know that while you cannot administer acupuncture to yourself, acupressure and EFT is a different story. You have nothing to lose by trying it either as you can find free books (remember those big buildings called libraries with all the free books) as well as free YouTube videos that will teach you everything you need to learn to practice yourself.

The videos and books specifically on the subject will be much more in depth but to keep in line with the spirit of this book, I will go over five specific points for water retention which massaging and tapping can help release. Note, there is no need to use all the points if you are short or time, just one or two a few times a day will suffice.

Sea of Energy - The sea of energy is located directly below the belly button. It is about two finger widths. Working on this point doesn't just relieve water retention but also helps treat chronic diarrhea, gas and constipation.

Shady Side of the Mountain - This is located on the inside part of the leg right below the knee and underneath the bone's large bulge. This is not just for treating water retention but can also be used for knee problems, leg tension, swelling, varicose veins and cramps.

Three Yin Crossing – This is located four finger widths above the inner anklebone on the back inner border of the shinbone. This acupressure point is for relieving edema. Caution: Do not stimulate this point during the eighth and ninth months of pregnancy.

Illuminated Sea – The Illuminated Sea is located one thumb width below the inside of the anklebone. It is not just for relieving water retention but also for swollen ankles

Blazing valley – Finally, the Blazing Valley is located on the middle of the arch of the foot midway between the outer tip of the big toe and the back of the heel.

Once you identify each point use prolonged finger pressure directly on the point; gradual, steady, penetrating pressure for approximately three minutes is ideal. Although you may be tempted to massage or rub the entire area, it is best just to hold the point steadily with direct finger pressure. The rule of thumb is to apply slow, firm pressure on the point at a ninety degree angle from the surface of the skin. If you are pulling the skin, then the angle of pressure is incorrect.

Consciously and gradually direct the pressure into the center of the part of the body you are working on. It's important to apply and release finger pressure gradually because this allows the tissues time to respond. The better your concentration as you move your fingers slowly into and out of the point, the more effective the treatment will be.

Avoid practicing acupressure right before a big meal or on a full stomach; wait until at least an hour after eating a light meal and even longer after eating a heavy meal. Avoid iced drinks (especially during the winter months), because extreme cold generally weakens your system and can counteract the benefits of acupressure. A cup of hot herbal tea would be good after an acupressure session along with a period of deep relaxation.

To wrap things up, as with every weight loss technique in this book - acupuncture, acupressure and EFT are tools in your toolbox. As the saying goes, take what you like and leave the rest. I've given you the information and while these protocols don't work for everyone, just remember that it is rare to find one thing that does (when we do we call it the cure).

I'm not suggesting that any of these three methods are the cure or sole modality for losing weight but hopefully I've given you enough evidence that it can indeed play some part in helping you meet your goals. Unless you try it, for all you know you could be in the camp that it does work for – and then that would be awesome! So if you are looking to exhaust every option and want to cover all your bases, give these puppies a shot.

CHAPTER 10

EXERCISE AND WATER RETENTION

Have you ever racked your brain to make sense of how you can seemingly exercise your butt off day in and day out, then step on the scale only to see no weight loss, or even worse, weight gain? No, you're not living in an alternate universe, and no, there's not some higher being out there whose sole existence is to drive you crazy. I swear there is a perfectly good explanation for why this happens.

An intense workout, especially one that involves heavy weight lifting and not enough recovery time (e.g. Crossfit, army style bootcamps, HIIT), can cause the body to retain water because water is attending to those muscles that are working overtime. Strengthening muscles or muscles that have been pulled or torn are areas where water travels to in order to heal.

You see, strength training causes microscopic tears in your muscle fibers. When these tears heal, the body rebuilds the muscles stronger than before. After a tough workout, blood rushes to the affected muscles to provide the nutrients that they need for recovery and to clear lactic acid and other cellular waste. The extra fluid causes muscles to become inflamed and the post-workout swelling usually begins almost immediately after a workout and can last three to seven days.

This means if you are one of those people doing hardcore workouts seven day a week with no rest day to speak of, your body will perpetually be in a post-workout swelling state. It's no wonder people who engage in these programs complain of bloating and puffiness on the level of the Stay Puft Marshmallow man.

Another way exercise can lead to weight gain is as a result of significant muscle gain. Muscle is comprised of small dense fibers while fat is comprised of larger, less dense droplets. This means that even if you lose fat, if you're simultaneously gaining muscle (common in people new to exercise and also known in the fitness community as newbie gains), you may notice weight gain.

Yet another culprit for weight gain as a result of exercise – or the wrong kind of exercise - is stress. There's no denying the aforementioned types of high intensity workouts put a high amount of stress on the body. Contrary to the popular mindset of those who support such workouts, pushing your body too much beyond its limits often actually does more harm than good.

The risk of injury aside, a workout environment that doesn't know the meaning of limitations can create a perfect storm for a significant stress response in your body. When this happens your adrenal glands increases production of cortisol which in turn causes an increase in blood pressure and leads to increased retention of sodium and fluid.

Does the answer to avoiding such swelling and weight gain then lie in copious amounts of hardcore cardio, like spinning, rowing or sprinting? Not exactly. On the other side of the coin, if you do too much high intensity or chronic cardio, e.g. two-hour treadmill sessions, you can put just as much stress on the body as you would with heavy resistance training.

If high intensity, heavy weight lifting and cardio are not the answer, should you just skip working out altogether? Wishful thinking! Just as there are exercises that lead to building muscle and have the unfortunate side effect of water retention from too much stress on the body, there are others that decrease stress, won't constantly tear muscle or lead to muscle gain, prevent water weight gain, and will assist you in shedding any water retention you may be carrying. Let's go over them now.

Vinyasa Yoga

If there is any workout program that does a great job lowering stress levels it's yoga and its focus on the mind-body connection, breathing and relaxation similar to meditation. Yoga postures have the ability to counter water retention in the different parts of the body such as legs, feet, abdomen, etc., and many of the twisting poses are all about aiding in digestion, which encourages the elimination of wastes.

The problem is that yoga in general is not a huge calorie burning exercise, which is still important if you want to lose as much weight as possible while firming up.

That being said out of the many types of yoga, two specific forms stand out from the crowd and align nicely with the scope of this book. These two practices are perfect for respectively getting a good calorie burn without having to deal with the dreaded backlash of torn and inflamed muscles (vinyasa) and sweating out water weight (hot yoga).

As I mentioned before, most yoga classes are painfully slow and easy, with the focus being on gentle stretching, or holding a position for a long time. Obviously, such movements – or lack thereof - are not going to generate a lot of heat, sweat or calorie burn. I have honestly emerged from yoga sessions where I didn't break a sweat, and felt like I had skipped the workout for a one-hour cool down.

The saving grace for anyone wanting to actually burn calories is vinyasa yoga, also called flow yoga, due to its fast paced fitness approach involving constant movement and challenging poses. The mix of cardio and isometric work which isn't designed to build muscle (poses focus on balancing and supporting your own body weight) which ensures you will not see any hypertrophy gains that could translate to weight gain from muscle mass or water retention.

On top of the fact that breaking a sweat is inevitable if you put in the work in a vinyasa class, which means you'll see some water weight loss, the constant movement can also allow bloat-causing gasses to pass out of the body.

Hot Yoga

Often associated with the style devised by Bikram Choudhury, hot yoga is now used to describe any number of yoga styles that use heat to increase an individual's flexibility in the poses. Some forms of hot yoga include Bikram yoga, Forrest yoga, Power yoga, Moksha Style Hot Yoga, and Tribalance yoga, so be on the lookout for classes being advertised under any of these names, as they will all serve your purpose.

The two most popular forms of yoga that you will probably find in your neighborhood are Bikram and Power Yoga, with Bikram being the most widely known form of hot yoga performed comprised of twenty-six poses performed in the same sequence for ninety minutes.

Hot yoga comes in second behind vinyasa as the highest calorie burning type of yoga with an average 330 calories burned for women and 460 calories burned for men per session according to a study published in Time Inc. Right off that bat that makes it a good exercise for weight loss purposes. However, hot yoga has another benefit that should make it an automatic go-to exercise for dropping weight fast.

With hot yoga, which is yoga performed in a room heated to approximately 105 degrees Fahrenheit with 40 percent humidity, you are going to sweat - buckets. Opening those sweat glands meets the criteria for one of the proven ways to relieve water retention and get the scale moving in the direction you want it to go.

Yogis who weigh themselves before and after a single hot yoga class usually notice a difference of one to three pounds, most of which represents water loss. As a result, instructors encourage students to hydrate themselves with about a quart of water two hours before class and to rehydrate generously after class to replace lost fluids.

Despite the fact that you will sweat a lot and burn a good amount of calories in a hot yoga class, there is a fine line that you need to toe or risk a most undesirable outcome – water weight gain.

There is such a thing as too much of a good thing and that applies here as well. It is common for people who throw themselves into aggressive hot yoga challenges, such as practicing daily for thirty or sixty days, or doing double ninety minute sessions in one day, to experience noticeable weight gain (ten to twenty pounds).

After all we've learned, all the reasons you might suspect results to backfire are probably right – too much time spent exercising in high temperatures (and yes, three hours would be considered too much) is a huge shock to the system and puts tremendous stress on the body.

Overdoing these classes (e.g. doing the 30 or 60 day daily practice) is not necessary or advisable. Think about it, would you hang out in a sauna for ninety minutes every single day for 30 or 60 days? Of course you wouldn't. So, why would you do that with hot yoga? Two to three times a week is enough, and the rest in between will do your body good.

Please note, if you are brand new to hot yoga or have taken significant time off from your practice, do not attempt this exercise right before your event or weigh in. Give yourself at least three days of leeway. If you have a few weeks of prep time start as far in advance as possible to acclimate to exercising in heat and allowing your body to balance itself out. For last minute, down to the wire prep, pure water weight reduction from sitting in the sauna would be a better bet than attempting to lose water weight from hot yoga – this is just one of the better exercises to do in the interim.

Another reason to be careful with hot yoga is that your body will lose salt and minerals through sweating as well as consuming a lot of water (which you'll want to do because dehydration is another cause of water retention) so in defense it will hang on to all the sodium in your blood and that can lead to water retention.

As a result, you *must* replenish your electrolytes with potassium, calcium, magnesium and sodium. Be sure to also drink four to six ounces of some type of electrolyte enhanced water every thirty or so minutes during your session and afterward as well as try to avoid wild swings in the amount of salt you normally consume otherwise be prepared for some serious bloat.

Thumping / Tapping Exercises

Body temperature is the foundation of good health. Like a fever, a low body temperature is a strong indicator that there is something wrong. One common side effect of low body temperature is fluid retention and easy weight gain. When low temperatures are normalized symptoms of fluid retention often disappear. So how do you do that? One option is to address the thyroid.

The link between the thyroid, low body temperature and fluid retention goes something like this: Low thyroid function can lead to low temperatures and low temperatures can cause fluid retention or bloating, tight rings, swollen ankles, and puffy face and eyes. Luckily, this is fixable by cutting off the problem at the head by addressing the thyroid.

Before you wage war on your thyroid, the first thing you will want to do is make sure the root of your problem is in fact low thyroid function, which is possible by assessing your body temperature. You could also get tests done by doctors, but this way is cheap, immediate and simple.

To test yourself for an under active thyroid, keep an electronic thermometer by your bed at night. When you wake up in the morning, place the thermometer in your armpit and hold it there for about ten minutes. Keep still and quiet. Any movement of the body can upset your temperature reading. Temperature of the body rises when you begin moving around. A temperature of 97.5°F. or lower is indicative of an under active thyroid. Keep a temperature log for five days. Menstruating women should perform test on second, third, and fourth day of menstruation.

If your readings are consistently low it (reflecting a low body temperature) and you are experiencing water retention it is time to get to work on normalizing your body. Really any exercise will help enhance thyroid function, so you want to make sure you are moving about throughout the day (walking, standing up instead of sitting down, climbing stairs instead of staking the elevator, stretching, etc.). However, specific thyroid exercises not too many people know about also can be done to stimulate the thyroid.

One such way to stimulate the thyroid manually, which has the added benefit of increasing the metabolism, is thymus tapping. This is done by thumping or tapping on your thymus gland (breastbone, center, over the heart) just down from the thyroid, but not the thyroid. The thymus is located behind the third rib, but any vibrations along the length of the upper sternum will stimulate it. Tapping the thymus stimulates immunity, loosens impacted toxins in the lungs, and stimulates the heart.

To do it, first take a couple of deep, relaxing breaths. Next, using your fingertips, knuckles in a gentle fist, or side of your fist, tap up and down about two to three inches along your sternum, between and above your mammary glands. The tapping should be a firm and gentle style of tapping - simulating the actual heartbeat. Thump for fifteen to twenty seconds and continue to take regular slow breaths. Practice this one to three times a day.

Another area to tap is the spleen neurolymphatic reflex points, located one rib below the breasts (below the bra line) directly under the nipples. This reduces chronic fatigue, provides an energy lift, help metabolize and detoxify the lymphatic system, balances blood chemistry levels and balances blood sugar levels within the pancreas. Both of these methods are widely used with those who practice energy work.

Alongside tapping, other exercises that can be done to really target your thyroid problem and get the blood flowing again can be found in yoga. Chin tucking poses such as halasana (plow pose) and sarvangasana (shoulder stand) are particularly effective for low thyroid problems because they compress and then released it allowing for better circulation. Another particularly helpful pose involves standing on your head with the chin tucked while humming and thumping both sides of the trachea.

Some additional poses good you may wish to include are: dhanurasa (bow pose), matsyasana (fish pose), sinhasana (lion pose), ustrasana (camel pose), shashankasana (hare pose), and ijjayi pranama (ocean breath) in your routine as they will also help.

For examples of any of the following poses gaiamtv.com has great tutorials (complete with pictures, step by step instructions and modifications). Simply put "gaiamtv poses" in your search engine and look for any of the specific poses listed above. Of course, there are plenty of other resources and videos available online for each and every single one of these poses as well.

Lastly, if you would like a whole comprehensive workout program to follow that targets your thyroid, check out Kundalini yoga. It is quite popular for breathing, arm and head movements that stimulate the thyroid. If you choose to try this route practice Kundalini Yoga on a daily basis with a strong focus on fifth chakra exercises and a little of the six chakra work here and there.

Steady State Cardio

We've already established chronic cardio and high intensity cardio are not the best choices for exercises that fend off water weight due to the toll on the muscles and stress to the body. However, low to moderate intensity steady state cardio, such as brisk walks or slow jogs anywhere from forty-five minute to one hour are perfectly fine. Exercises with a low perceived rate of effort, such as the ones I've suggested won't cause a major shock to your system, requiring tremendous recovery time, or elevate cortisol, but will burn lots of calories.

To be clear, I have nothing inherently against high intensity cardio workouts and think they are great for certain people under certain circumstances. For example, if your goal were to maximize your cardiovascular endurance, improve speed and agility, and lose weight without a specific deadline (applicable if you had a lot of weight to lose) then high intensity interval training (a heart rate between 90-100% of your maximum) paired with adequate rest time would be a fine plan.

You can torch a lot of calories and maintain or build up a good amount of muscle, which allows you to burn slightly more calories throughout the day just existing. There's also something called the after burn effect, which basically means your metabolism is raised a little longer (you continue burning calories) after an intense workout while your body gets back to normal – something that doesn't happen with low/moderate steady state cardio.

Provided you were eating properly (low carb, moderate fat and protein, and low salt) along with drinking enough water, you would keep water retention at bay and lose weight at a slow and steady pace.

However, when you have only a few days or weeks to make as big a change in your weight as possible (as the subtitle promises), how many calories you burn, your deficit and managing your water weight are all of the utmost importance. I've revealed the effects of high intensity workouts on water weight already, and here's how steady state cardio wins the battle of the deficit / calorie burn in the long run.

It's a proven fact that steady state cardio is bar none, the best type of exercise to burn actual *fat*, provided you remain in the fat burning zone (heart rate between 50-65%) for around an hour. In contrast, high intensity workouts burn primarily glucose (blood sugar) and glycogen (carbs stored in your muscles and liver for energy).

What happens when you do an intense workout when you are deficient in carbohydrates (glucose and glycogen) because you've restricted your carb intake – as you should be if you want to drop the pounds quickly? Well, your body being the ever-resourceful survivor that it is turns to other sources to produce glucose, such as amino acids or muscle tissue.

In other words, if you're not getting a lot of carbs and eating in a deficit but still working out like a madman/woman at your box (slang for crossfit gyms), your body is going to burn away your muscle tissue to allow you to continue working out at that intensity while being more prone to injury. Less muscle leads to a lowered metabolism and less overall calories burned, and if you injure yourself that means even less calories will be burned.

On the other hand, when you do long steady state cardio you might burn the same amount of calories as a shorter higher intensity workout (it'll just take longer), and you won't find yourself out of commission from injury or a sore body that needs a few days to recover. You can do your steady state cardio daily, and even pair it with sweat suits or other methods listed in the book without risk. The result? More targeted fat loss, more calories burned, less muscle spared.

Again, I have to stress that this is the best strategy when you need to lose a lot of weight fast paired with the fact that you will need to be on a low carb/low calorie diet while working out. This combination of diet and exercise is to be done for a short duration - no more than a few weeks at most.

A more long term and balanced approach would be to combine resistance training and moderate intensity cardio three to four times a week while eating at a calorie deficit no more than a twenty percent your TDEE (total daily energy expenditure), or if your aesthetic and fitness goals warrant it, a high intensity training program while eating at a calorie level suitable to fuel those types of workouts.

Cardio Twist

So far we know cardio and certain types of yoga are the ideal ways to train for rapid water weight loss in a short period of time as both exercises won't build too much muscle or overstress the body, resulting in swelling/bloating. Additionally, both exercises will burn a lot of calories and fat as opposed to glycogen, and are mild enough to not pose a threat of injury, permitting you to train daily without needing to take precious days off for recovery.

Now, obviously you could piecemeal your program together and do well, but if you are the type of person who would prefer to just have a succinct program neatly bundled together for you, here is where CardioTwist comes into play.

Cardio Twist is a one-hour workout DVD by yours truly that blends the best yoga poses for releasing fluid retention (e.g. twisting, chin to neck, etc.) with cardio movements to create a continuous workout flow. Your heart rate will be elevated the entire time so you are ensured a substantial calorie burn, but remain in the cardiovascular range so that you tap into fat stores as opposed to glycogen. The workout was designed to also meet the other requirements that make these ideal workouts as I've reviewed in the opening paragraph to this section.

Again, this is not mandatory for you to purchase in order to see success in the program, but it will make it easier for some of you who want to remove the guesswork and fuss involved in putting together your own regimen from scratch. If you are interested in purchasing the DVD, which is to be released in April, you may do so directly from my website www.thighgaphack.com/cardiotwist if you are reading this after April 2015, or email me at camille@thighgaphack.com to be alerted first once the DVD becomes available.

Swimming

If you love the water you are in luck because the next recommended exercise to accompany your diet plan for losing water weight fast is swimming or doing exercise movements in the deep water.

There are many pros to swimming. First, water pressure can force water out of the body's tissues and push the body to eliminate through urination. That's an easy one or two pounds in water weight loss there. However, make sure that you drink additional water after a long or strenuous swim, as chlorinated or salted water can cause dehydration.

Beyond water weight, swimming uses almost all the major muscle groups, and places a vigorous demand on your heart and lungs while being easy on the joints, thus reducing the risk of injury. It develops muscle strength and endurance, and improves posture and flexibility. Additionally, it's ideal for people with injuries or for those who carry so much weight that they find walking and other forms of exercise painful.

It can burn a lot of calories and truly be a great form of exercise - the operative word here being *can*. Don't be fooled into thinking submerging yourself in the water and simply doing a few laps or splashing around fits the bill – that does not a workout make.

To burn calories on par with other exercises with swimming you will need to maintain a level of intensity equivalent to jogging or brisk walking where holding a conversation is difficult - or a heart rate of seventy to eighty percent of it's maximum, for around forty-five minute to an hour. To estimate your target rate, subtract your age from 220 and multiply by 0.8. To ensure you're staying in the zone, stop after every ten to fifteen laps and use the pool clock to count your pulse for six seconds; tack a zero onto the number.

To be honest, this is difficult for most untrained swimmers to accomplish and so, along with factors like buoyancy dragging your overall calorie burning down, you might not be getting as much of a workout as you think you are.

Wait, so am I recommending swimming or not? I totally am, but probably not in the way you were thinking of before (a few laps around the pool). If you are going to use swimming for weight loss and aren't trained enough to do vigorous swimming for long period of time, here are some things you will definitely want to do:

First, get yourself a kickboard, hand paddle, swim fins, and/or foam buoys that fit between your legs. Most pools have them, but you can also buy your own at a local sporting goods store. If using a toy that occupies your arms be sure to really activate the larger muscles in your legs by kicking them intensely when you swim; if the toy/aid goes on your feet to keep you a float thereby freeing your arms, work those free arms as much as possible with large strokes.

Alternate laps where you go as fast as you can with laps where you swim more slowly to catch your breath. Rest less by making sure no more than ten percent of your water time is spent loitering in your lane. Try to pause no more than ten seconds between laps or intervals.

Finally, and this is probably the easiest option for most people, try water based activities and classes like aqua aerobics, shallow water walking and deep-water running wearing a flotation vest. Heck, you can even incorporate all of the above to make up your one hour work out and you will be guaranteed to leave having scorched a ton of calories.

If you don't see yourself successfully being able to do the above every time you step into the pool to get your work out, I would recommend swimming as a supplement to other workout plans mentioned here (yoga, steady state cardio, etc.).

Whether you add swimming to your repertoire or focus on using it solely for exercise, know that swimming in a pool may be more conducive to the type of workout you're looking for than swimming at a beach or lake; pools often have lap swim hours, and you won't have to contend with rolling waves or boats.

One thing to be mindful of though is that studies have shown that swimming in cold water leads to an increased appetite which could make sticking to your diet extremely difficult and complete wiping out any benefits of swimming as a weight loss tool. As a result, make sure that whatever water you swim in is close to temperature of a heated swimming pool (approximately eighty degrees Fahrenheit or twenty seven degrees Celsius).

Mini Trampoline or Rebounding

We've covered the lymphatic system and its role in the water retention fight numerous times already. If you will recall lymphatic flow requires muscular contraction from exercise and movement, gravitational pressure and internal massage to the valves of lymph ducts.

While generally any exercise in which you do a lot of movement will have an effect on pumping the fluid by meeting the muscular contraction from exercise requirement, one exercise in particular takes the cake for stimulating your system by meeting all three methods – rebounding or jumping on a therapeutic mini trampoline.

Rebounding is reported to increase lymph flow by a whopping fifteen to thirty times. That is because vertical motion workouts such as rebounding are much different and much more beneficial and efficient than horizontal motion workouts, such as jogging or running. For example, only twenty minutes of rebounding is the equivalent to one hour of running for a cardiovascular workout.

But wait, there's more - rebounding reduces your body fat; firms your legs, thighs, abdomen, arms, and hips; increases your agility; and improves your sense of balance. It strengthens your muscles overall, provides an aerobic effect for your heart, rejuvenates your body when it's tired, and generally puts you in a state of health and fitness without attracting fluid accumulation under the skin.

On top of all of that, it also stimulates your digestion, allowing foods to evacuate faster and improves metabolism. The steady bounce sets up a pulsating rhythm transmitted by the nervous system to the brain area responsible for regulating the intestinal system, which reestablishes one's rhythmical bowel activity. Metabolism is improved because all your other organ systems are being recharged. If your body is working, no doubt your metabolism will follow.

Finally, jumping on a rebounder is remarkably gentle on the joints. There's no solid ground to suddenly stop the bouncing of your feet so your movements are perfectly safe, and they make the effect of gravity beneficial.

To reap all the benefits of this amazing exercise, the first thing you'll need is a rebounder. You can either purchase one to use in the comfort of your own home, or you can opt to find a rebounding fitness class, which has become more popular in recent years.

If you go the fitness class route, take your pick from boutique companies like JumpLife, which pairs rebounding with the atmosphere of a nightclub complete with strobe lights and club music, to offerings from huge workout chains like Crunch gym, 24 Hour Fitness and Bally's Total Fitness, where the more classic group class dynamic is available.

If you would rather not have to deal with membership dues and the like, you can find rebounders and mini-trampolines for any price point at websites like Amazon, or any of the big box retailers like Target, Wal-Mart or Sears. You might be able to get a more quality unit for a much cheaper price if you search on

Craigslist or EBay. There are tons of people out there unloading their barely used exercise equipment for various reasons, from moving to de-cluttering to simply failing to stick to their exercise regimen.

Once you've gotten your equipment and laced up your sneakers (do not rebound barefoot) you can either buy rebounding workout DVD's or find free workout videos online for a set routine, or you can follow the following three basic rebounding exercises to start:

The Health Bounce is gently bouncing up and down on a rebounder without your feet leaving the mat. It is very low impact and very effective at moving your lymphatic system. Most folks can easily do this for an hour or more while watching TV.

The Strength Bounce is jumping as high as you can. It strengthens primary and stabilizer muscles throughout your body, improves your balance, and moves your lymphatic system like nothing else. That's what you want to work up to.

Aerobic Bouncing is jumping jacks, twisting, running in place, bouncing on one leg at a time, dancing, and any other crazy maneuvers you can think of. Doing these high intensity aerobic exercises will get your blood pumping and your sweat on. Again, just fifteen to twenty minutes is all you really need to get the job done.

274

CHAPTER 11

CARB REFEEDS

In what is likely to be your favorite chapter in this entire book, it is time to talk about refeeds, better known in the fitness world as carb refeeds. I have saved this for last because if you have made it all this way you deserve to be rewarded with good news.

It is no secret that carbs taste good - so good that many people overeat them - which is why it's a sound move to consciously diminish the amount of carbs you consume while trying to shed weight. Well, that and the other handful of reasons I've discussed, such as the role carbs play in the body retaining more water, blocking fat burning and stoking the appetite.

One thing that carbs are undeniably good at though is providing the body with energy. Every now and then when dieting or weight loss stalls out, such a boost comes with what many would call unexpected benefits. This is the reason we carb reefed.

Carb refeeds are just what they sound like: a chance to ease up on your carb restriction for a short time. Doing so gives a shot of jolt to your metabolism, reduces cortisol, refills muscle glycogen, restores hormones, prevents an overly catabolic environment, and restores leptin levels in the dieter reduced as a result of caloric restriction. With lower leptin comes increased hunger and reduced adherence to a diet. Cravings arise, energy wanes, and immunity suffers. The lack of leptin elicits the cascade of hormones that down regulate metabolism and energy expenditure.

Your muscles use less energy and become more efficient – but weaker and less effective. Menstruation and fertility become issues. Dropping calories even more just makes the problem worse. You need to restore leptin periodically to right the path. A carb refeed can help you achieve this.

Before we get into the specifics on how to successfully go about a carb reefed please note that it is not right for everyone (obese individuals) and the length of your reefed really depends on your current body fat. Refeeds work best for men who have fifteen percent body fat and women with around twenty percent body fat. For very obese people, you probably do not need to do a carb reefed but could get away with one every two weeks. For very lean individuals, once every three or so days seems optimal. For everyone else (most people) once a week is best.

To get into what refeeding actually entails, I hate to burst your bubble, but it is not a free pass to run to the nearest bakery and stuff your face with pastries. Carb choices should consist primarily of glucose-based starches without resorting to grain consumption or sugar.

Examples of ideal foods are potatoes, rice, pasta and bread. Technically any low sugar carb source will work, e.g. low fat crackers and chips, waffles or pancake – but I don't want you activating those taste buds if you can help it. The main thing is to keep sugar and fruit low (eighty percent glucose and twenty percent sucrose is recommended) as this has all the benefits you are looking for.

Additionally, you will want to keep potassium high while protein, fat and fiber are kept constant to low. As for how many carbs you should consume, since you should be relatively low carb anyway (50 – 100 grams), you can get away with doubling it.

If you keep protein and fat constant, yes, your calories will be much higher than usual. That's the point! Your metabolism will greatly benefit though, and once you go back to low carbs/calories, you will find yourself burning more calories without any extra work on your part, but by nature of your higher metabolism.

Carb refeeds that are done right will leave you feeling disinterested in food. This shows that your body has had enough and doesn't crave any more food or carbohydrates. Of course, the main indicator that you have done a proper refeed is weight loss. The refeed will have the effect of pulling water outside of the muscle cell into the muscle cell. Along with increased muscle glycogen, this will give you a lean appearance the next day, ideally also causing the much anticipated whoosh effect we spoke about earlier. To take advantage of this overnight weight loss it might behoove you to schedule your final refeed the night before you need to look your best.

For an even leaner look, you can opt to do a dry carb feed by limiting water intake. The downside is that you will end up feeling very thirsty and probably miserable. Therefore, you might want to save this strategy towards the very end of your plan if you choose to implement this tweaked version of carb loading at all.

Lastly, I don't recommend this, but some people have had success with creating the whoosh effect by drinking alcohol (doesn't this chapter just keep on getting better?) during their carb refeed since alcohol is a mild diuretic. Keep in mind though that alcohol only in the form of spirits are allowed as sweet drinks are forbidden. In other words, wine, beer and cosmos are out of the question.

CHAPTER 12

ENDING THE PLAN

You have read the book, stuck to your diet, carb loaded (refeed), pounded and then rationed the water, pushed through the exercise, and boosted your progress with the other various techniques and tools offered within these pages. You've transformed your body by dropping an incredible amount of water weight and even some fat, zipped into your amazing outfit, and wowed everyone or met your target weight goal for your weigh in, competition, video/photo shoot gig.

Congratulations on a job well done, and in only a matter of weeks to boot! I'd say you are now something of a pro when it comes to manipulating your physique in a smart and strategic manner – probably even more than the so-called professional fitness folks. Unfortunately, this can be just as much of a bad thing as a good thing. Let me explain why.

After everything is said and done one of three things may occur. The first is the ideal outcome, which is that you are enamored with your new weight loss and will want to keep it going by continuing the processes it took to get you to your new physique.

My hope is that you heed my warning and switch over to more balanced and healthy tactics to continue your progress and go on to see steady weight loss over the course of time. Some of you will do just that and make me proud by sending me your updates (I welcome them with open arms) of your exciting journey into a completely revamped lifestyle, but this will not be the narrative for everyone.

Being a professional at cutting weight can be a detriment because once you've succeeded at quick weight loss, you become confident in knowing that you can do it again whenever you'd like. It may seem like a good thing to have confidence in your abilities and knowledge, but it can also be a double edge sword that erases any sense of urgency or necessity to revamp your lifestyle. That goes for either avoiding a return to old junk foods and lack of exercise or stopping the extreme dieting and exercise meant for short-term use only in this book.

It is not uncommon for people to feel exempt from having to resort to following the normal rhetoric and rules of diet and exercise after quickly losing weight with hacks and shortcuts. They get an inflated sense that the regular rules don't apply to them as much anymore because they are now privy to the fast acting, lesser known, secret world of weight loss manipulation, which in their mind can be wielded at a moments notice.

In practice, it's not so cut and dry. Every time you gain and lose the same pounds over again it's a struggle. One might think the willpower is strengthened or that it would be easier each time, but in fact the opposite is true. Entering the damaging and unhealthy pattern of yo-yo dieting can take a large toll on your self-esteem, mental health and last but not lease, body.

People tend to beat themselves up for undoing all their progress (even if they were compliant in doing so), wonder what's the point of losing the weight to gain it all again sooner or later, or delay restarting the weight loss program indefinitely because it's much easier to not do anything.

Hopefully you see how the initial belief of impunity from the tenets of balanced and moderate dieting and exercise can result in reckless behavior, habits and patterns that even with all these tricks, are difficult to overcome and yield undesirable chains of events to occur.

An equally unfortunate but common scenario once you finish your dieting period is feeling compelled or entitled to overeat after weeks of putting your body through the rigor and with no upcoming event driving your motivation. This is not so much a deliberate act to eat with abandon because you can always bounce back as the attitude we've just covered.

In fact, it may start out innocent enough - perhaps you initially just plan on one indulgent meal or two, but things quickly snowball out of control and before you know it you are straight back at square one, except you got there faster and possibly put on even more weight than before. This can be explained by the real changes your body undergoes – e.g. when you lose weight, your metabolism slows or when you suddenly increase carbs all the bloat comes rushing back.

What's more is that binging – even on tasty junk foods – will leave you feeling really bad. What will happen is all that food will just end up sitting in your shrunken stomach making you feel bloated and tired. This is because in order to digest the food, the body pulls blood away from your muscles to your stomach. A lot of food will take longer to digest, leaving you feeling pretty bad, which is the opposite of what you are attempting to do by gorging on the off limit foods post plan.

I say all of this to say that instead of what you have accomplished empowering you to move forward towards a healthier lifestyle, the shortcuts and fast acting tips handicap you because you rely on them as a crutch you can always lean on when you fall off the wagon or you don't come off the plan as advised and spiral down the binge eating rabbit hole.

On the other spectrum, but equally as ill advised, some of you will love your results so much that you just won't want to stop employing the tactics that are working so well for you despite my warnings. So you will continue going to the sauna, getting colonics too regularly, eating a low calorie diet, exercising daily, intermittent fasting, etc.

As stated before, this is *not* recommended as the protocols in this book is specifically not a long-term weight loss plan. Such stressors are not meant to be sustainable and will eventually take a negative toll on your health in the form of decreased muscles, energy, metabolism, and wacky hormones, which can lead to all kinds of serious mental and physical illnesses and problems.

Obviously, all of these terrible outcomes but the first one mentioned can be avoided if you have the right attitude about the objective and limitations of this plan and commit to coming off of it properly. So, what's the best way to transition over to a more healthy and balanced weight loss program?

First things first, get a firm end date in mind. For most people the natural end date will be the day after your special event or weigh in. Working backwards from there, make sure that you do not exceed four weeks maximum if you plan to be a little more conservative in the protocols you choose or have less weight to lose, and no more than two weeks if you plan to aggressively attach your weight loss by combining multiple tactics or have a lot of weight to lose.

Along with a concrete timeline, you should also have a specific number of pounds you want to lose. A weight objective benchmark will be more useful at blocking the temptation to continue dieting and losing weight beyond your original goal.

If you don't hit the goal in the time frame (maximum of 30 days) because you chose to go a more conservative route, didn't give yourself enough time or didn't have enough weight to lose (the skinnier you are the less weight will come off) still stop and transition over to more moderate eating and exercising to give your body a rest.

When ending the plan one of the most important things you should do is still continue to rehydrate. Not with soda, juice, beer, or coffee, but plain, unsweetened water. It is imperative to keeping up the good habits like drinking lots of water, which will keep phantom hunger at bay, and only eat when you are hungry (which you should now really be able to identify, as well as thirst). The added benefit of drinking water is it will help you avoid the urge to chow down immediately.

While I mentioned calories need to be raised, it is of the utmost importance that you don't just jump straight into adding 300+ calories to your diet. Each week increase your intake by one hundred calories or so. You will want to stop adding calories once you've brought your calorie deficit up to no more than twenty percent of your TDEE (total daily energy expenditure).

A gradual increase of carbs may be included in your increased calorie allotment each week as well but it should not be in the form of simple carbs. Remember, if you are still looking to maintain or lose real fat, you can't eat anything, but you can eat more of the wholesome nutritious foods you were eating before while following this intense cutting program.

Slowly increasing your carbs and/or overall intake will lead to more energy without overloading your stomach, so while you may reduce your workouts from every day down to four to five per week, keep up the cardio to avoid fat accumulation. Many people make the mistake of taking a week off, which turns into two, then three, etc.

Remember, cardio will prevent the glycogen stores from becoming overfilled by your increased carb intake while also adding in at least twenty minutes of resistance training before your cardio session. Please note, whether you go for light or heavy weights depends on your preferred physique.

To avoid inducing binging episodes, take the time to write out or devise meal plans so you know in advance exactly what you will consume for each meal in the day. Don't leave it to whimsy as avoiding sugar is of the utmost importance post diet.

Additionally, do not go grocery shopping immediately after coming off the diet, especially if you only done a program for less than two weeks (it takes about three weeks to form a habit). This doesn't mean starve to death. It means being prepared by having enough food stocked to last you a week or two after you end your plan (fresh foods will last for weeks and weeks if frozen), or give online grocery shopping/delivery a go.

Failing those options, only go shopping after you've eaten so you're not hungry and tempted to grab snacks or old comfort food staples, and bring a shopping list with just enough cash to purchase those items.

Finally, make a pact with yourself that you will refrain from doing another drastic cut or any of the hardcore quick water weight loss strategies in the book for at least three of four months after you've given your body a rest, with the exception of intermittent fasting.

You shouldn't need to resort to that anyway if you maintain your losses and steadily implement sound dieting and exercise guidelines. However, should you find yourself putting on a little weight (more than likely water weight), don't panic. You can nip it in the bud right away without extreme rigidity.

Simply reevaluate your numbers to identify any potential errors in your determined BMR (again, it decreases once you lose weight), TDEE and/or the amount of calories you are eating. The easiest ways to accomplish this is to buy a food scale, physical activity tracker, and enter your updated numbers into a

BMR calculator. Since everything is based on these numbers, it is imperative that they are accurate.

There is nothing wrong with taking stock and readjusting if need be. If after three to four months of regular dieting and training, you find the need to go for another round of heavy or mild cutting by turning to this book, by all means - go ahead. Your body will have sufficiently recuperated from your first round and you should have even less weight (water and fat) to lose provided you judiciously made the transition as I have instructed.

CHAPTER 13

WHAT TO DO NOW

There you have it; everything you need to know to drastically shrink your body in as little time as possible by understanding and working with your body in the most efficient, and strategic ways possible. The only thing left for you to do is to pick and choose which techniques are a good fit, go forth and do the work.

While you are at it, may I suggest taking a few before pictures so that you can visibly see your progress? Research shows that this is one way people remain committed to their programs. I know the thought of collecting physical evidence reminding you of the road ahead may not seem appealing, but at the very least you can finally put those selfie skills you've honed to good use.

Generally, a front, side and back shot in as little clothes as you feel comfortable, so that you can really see the contour of the body, is best (e.g. sports bra and shorts for women or swim trunks for guys).

I am delighted that you took the time to read this, and I hope it has been informative, valuable and helpful to you. As I mentioned before, it pains me to see people cutting weight by putting their bodies in extreme danger just because it's too taboo for anyone to tackle the subject of water weight loss in a book. If you know me, I don't shy away from controversial subjects and I think shining a spotlight on something people will do regardless so that they can do it in a safer way is super important.

If you agree and would like to show your support or appreciation that someone has finally stepped up to tackle this subject comprehensively instead of it remaining a huge secret only privy to professional fitness professionals and competitors, I would ask for nothing more than for you to take a minute or two to share your honest opinion with others.

Nowadays with so many so-called experts trying to cash in on the fitness industry, it can be hard to separate the wheat from the chaff. As a result, readers like you must depend on other readers (like you) to determine whether a resource really contains the information he or she seeks before spending hard earned money on a product.

I can only hope you feel you have gotten the information you sought within the pages of this book. It's been a year in the making only because I did not want to leave anything out and I wanted to break everything down so that people located anywhere on the fitness spectrum (from newbies to seasoned pros) could benefit.

Lastly, if you have any unresolved questions about something in that book that you need clarification on, I encourage you to reach out to me. My direct email is Camille@thighgaphack.com. I am happy to help or just hear the success stories I'm sure you will have to share.

For those of you who have more in depth questions or feel like you need help beyond the scope of this book, I've taught thousands of people how to lose weight (fat, unwanted overdeveloped muscle, and water weight for special occasions) so they can finally get the results they want, and I can help you too. Again, you can email me directly to inquire about my consultant rates.

You may also want to check out my other books, *"The Thigh Gap Hack"*, and *"Bye-Bye Thunder Thighs"*, which deal with very common problem areas for women before diving into personal training/consulting.

Finally, as I've said time and time again, I love researching, talking and writing about fitness and always have my fingers on the pulse of new happenings.

I usually share my latest findings, research, success stories, tools and resources, and my favorite tips and tricks on fitness related topics (from fashion to food to gadgets and beyond) on my newsletter, which you can sign up for at http://www.thighgaphack.com, on my facebook page (www.facebook.com/thighgaphack), twitter page (www.twitter.com/thighgaphack), and last but not least, my youtube page (www.youtube.com/thighgaphack).

###

Prelude to 'The Skinny Bible' and 'Dump The Oil, Drop The Fat' (The Oil-Free Diet)

Have you ever read a book claiming to hold precious secrets and answers to a burning topic or question you are interested in, only to find common knowledge fare that's either outdated, not applicable to real life, or not nearly comprehensive enough?

I have, and it's downright insulting and infuriating! So, when I set out to write *'The Skinny Girl Bible'*, I wanted to make sure the content was so real, relevant, and encompassing that it would have no choice but to be called the downright authority on the non-obvious rules thin women live by.

With a name like The Skinny Girl Bible, I think it's evident that I won't be holding anything back. You won't find just ten or so actual nuggets (in other words a listacle padded enough to be disguised as a book) here.

What you will find is over 100 fresh *commandments* (hard and fast rules like in the real bible) expounded upon so you not only get to see the way many thin women think, but plan, act and react to certain scenarios that result in them easily

293

keeping the weight off. From page one, I jump straight to the point and there is so much to cover, you can rest assured that there is zero room for filler.

I chose this name for the book not only because it reflects a lack of brevity. The bible is the book of life, full of wise teachings, lessons and tenets that if followed will allow people to find happiness, peace and meaning in this world.

'The Skinny Girl Bible' has a similar objective: It is full of wise teachings and lessons from those who have successfully acquired what you want – confidence and happiness in their skin, and control over food that holds so many others captive, and gives you the step-by-step breakdown of how you can get it for yourself.

My fifth book, 'The Oil-Free Diet', is scheduled to be released around the same time as 'The Skinny Girl Bible' (about two weeks apart) and I'm super excited about this subject as it is a concept most people are unfamiliar with, but a tactic that is highly effective for weight loss.

As of this writing (2015), there are no books on how to successfully utilize an oil-free diet and that makes me incredulous. I have all but no choice but to pen this book on a subject only a select few fitness savvy people have ever even heard of and are benefiting greatly from.

Now, before you go all bonkers from the thought of dropping oil from your diet, you should know that an oil-free diet is not the same as a fat free diet. Fat is not inherently bad and you can eat foods with naturally occurring oil and fats (e.g. the fat that is naturally present in plant foods, nuts and animals, etc.).

There is however a big difference between the pure liquid fat we add to our diet in the form of processed oils, such as olive and vegetable oils, which have all of the good stuff stripped from it during processing, and oils and fats from whole foods with the vitamins in tact.

First of all, at 4,000 calories per pound (120 per tablespoon) oil is the most calorie dense food on the planet, topping *all* other food for calories per pound. Let that sink in for a little bit. It is pure fat and given the fact that many of you are currently feeling queasy at the mere thought of eliminating oil from your diet should tell you how addicting it is. However, it is probably one of the smallest changes you can make to your diet that makes losing weight as effortless as can be.

I'm aware the concept of an oil-free diet sounds impossible, but really it isn't. In the book I'll show you how to go oil-free without feeling like you are even on a diet (no, you won't have to give up on food tasting pleasurable), how to cook and bake without oil, the best oil free recipes, oil substitutions, how to eat out on the diet, etc. You'll also learn about all the additional benefits your body will experience besides weight loss on the diet.

If you know me by now and the topics I tend to gravitate towards, you would understand why I'm just the gal to blow the lid open on what will arguably be the next big dieting trend. I guarantee you that by the end of the book you'll be thanking me for introducing you to this unconventional dieting method that no one else is has had the foresight to explore.

As I've said before, I think of it as my duty to stay ahead of the dieting curves and bring you the latest/greatest and most effective methods to help you in your weight loss goals, and I'm really bringing my A-game with this one!

If you are interested in finding out more information about either of these books, and you know you are, I encourage you to head on over to my website, www.thighgaphack.com. Additionally, make sure you subscribe to my YouTube page www.youtube.com/thighgaphack, where I regularly make announcements, videos and run contests/giveaways relating to my latest books, to be kept in the loop.